# 2000–2001

# Nelson's Pocket Book of Pediatric Antimicrobial Therapy

FOURTEENTH EDITION

# 2000–2001

# Nelson's Pocket Book of Pediatric Antimicrobial Therapy

**FOURTEENTH EDITION**

**John D. Nelson, MD**
Professor Emeritus of Pediatrics
The University of Texas
Southwestern Medical Center
at Dallas
Southwestern Medical School
Dallas, Texas

**John S. Bradley, MD**
Director, Division of Infectious Diseases
Children's Hospital and Health Center,
San Diego
Associate Clinical Professor of Pediatrics
University of California, San Diego,
School of Medicine
San Diego, California

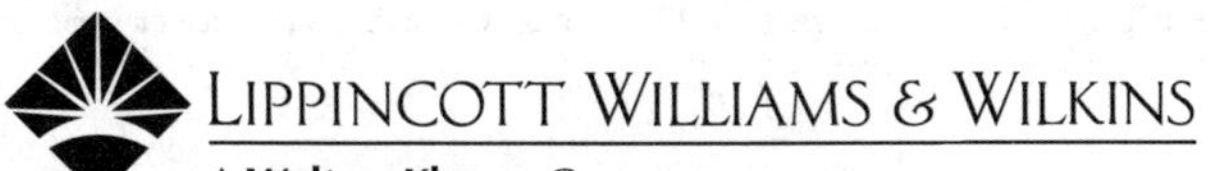


A **Wolters Kluwer** Company

Philadelphia • Baltimore • New York • London
Buenos Aires • Hong Kong • Sydney • Tokyo

*Editor:* Jonathan Pine
*Managing Editor:* Jennifer Kullgren
*Marketing Manager:* Adam Glazer
*Director of Manufacturing Operations:* Sue Cohen
*Assistant Production Manager:* Ruth Cruz
*Production Editor:* Kim Langford, Silverchair Science + Communications
*Cover Designer:* Brown Hornet Design, Inc.
*Compositor:* Silverchair Science + Communications
*Printer:* Vicks Lithograph & Printing


**227 East Washington Square**
**Philadelphia, PA 19106-3780 USA**
**LWW.com**



Printed in the USA

First Edition, 1975

**ISBN 0-781-72570-4**



99 00 01 02
1 2 3 4 5 6 7 8 9 10

## CONTENTS

# I. INTRODUCTION TO THE FOURTEENTH EDITION

I appreciate greatly the helpful criticisms and suggestions of my infectious disease colleagues at the University of Texas Southwestern Medical Center: Doctors Doug Hardy, Hasan Jafri, George McCracken, Ian Michelow, Octavio Ramilo, Violeta Rodriguez, and Jane Siegel. I extend special thanks to John Bennett for reviewing the antifungal section, to Pablo Sánchez for help with the newborn section, and to Peter Hotez for advice about the parasitic diseases section. Tammy Bratton, Pharm.D. and Gayle Romanowski, Pharm.D. provided invaluable information.

Recent editions of this book have been translated into Chinese, German, Greek, Indonesian, Italian, Polish, Portuguese, Russian, and Spanish. The task of the translators is complicated by the variability of drug availability in different countries. Fortunately, the major antimicrobials are universally available.

The large number of related drugs means that multiple options are available for a great many diseases. To avoid cluttering up and expanding the book, I have indicated only one or two options for treating most infections. Clearly, other regimens may be suitable.

Some dosages and indications differ from those in the manufacturers' package inserts. In such situations, the dosages recommended in this book have been found by controlled studies or by clinical experience to be efficacious and safe.

For more than 25 years, this book has been a solo exercise. Beginning with this fourteenth edition, the solo becomes a duet. My partner is John S. Bradley, M.D., who is Director of the Division of Infectious Diseases at Children's Hospital and Health Center in San Diego, California. I have known and admired his clinical and investigative expertise for years, but we have never worked together nor did he train with me. For these reasons and because he is a full generation younger than I am, he brings a fresh, vital viewpoint to the recommendations for selection of antimicrobial therapy. His daily involvement with direct patient care ensures a practical perspective.

Beginning with the fifteenth edition, Dr. Bradley will assume primary responsibility for the biennial revisions of this book. I am confident that I could not turn it over to more capable hands and mind.

John D. Nelson, MD

Since entering the field of pediatric infectious diseases in the late 1970s, I have been fortunate to be able to blend clinical practice, an incredibly rewarding endeavor for an infectious diseases specialist, with clinical investigation. It has been clear to me that the "art of antimicrobial therapy" is a blend of microbiology, pharmacology, clinical research on anti-infectives, and good clinical judgment for each individual patient. Of all the books available to give practical advice to clinicians on antimicrobial therapy for children, John Nelson's *Pocket Book of Pediatric Antimicrobial Therapy* has always been the most valuable, referencing in a portable format the antimicrobials, the organisms, and the clinical syndromes. Every student and resident who has taken a rotation in infectious diseases with us since 1981 has received a copy of Dr. Nelson's book. On hospital rounds or in the clinic, when the question of treatment is raised and a quick answer is not forthcoming, we always ask, "What does John Nelson say?" The student, resident, or attending with an opinion different from Dr. Nelson's should be prepared to defend his or her position!

Most of you probably have the same reaction as I have to Dr. Nelson's decision to begin to step down as the editor of his *Pocket Book*. He just can't do that! I have valued and used Dr. Nelson's advice for the past 20 years; my patients have received better care and I have become a better physician as a direct result of his advice. No one can replace John Nelson, and I will not attempt to do so. It will, however, be an honor and a privilege for me to learn from "the master" during the next editions of *Nelson's Pocket Book of Pediatric Antimicrobial Therapy*. I fully intend to uphold the philosophy of the practical nature of the book, which has made it so useful to me and everyone else involved in the care of children. Dr. Nelson has assured me, and this will be a comfort to everyone who uses this reference, that he will continue to co-edit the *Pocket Book* for many years to come!

As Dr. Nelson has noted with each edition, I, too, welcome suggestions from the users of the *Pocket Book* on how to improve it. John also keeps reminding me to keep it short!

John S. Bradley, MD

## II. CHOOSING AMONG AMINOGLYCOSIDES, BETA-LACTAMS, AND MACROLIDES

New drugs should be compared with others in the same class regarding (1) antimicrobial spectrum, (2) degree of potency within the spectrum, (3) pharmacokinetic and pharmacodynamic properties, (4) demonstrated efficacy in clinical trials, (5) tolerance, toxicity and side effects, and (6) cost. If there is no substantial benefit in any of those areas, one should opt for using an older, more familiar drug because of the risk of unexpected adverse effects inherent in any new product.

**Aminoglycosides.** Five aminoglycosidic antibiotics are available in the United States as major drugs for coliform bacillary and *Pseudomonas* infections: amikacin, gentamicin, kanamycin, netilmicin, and tobramycin. (Streptomycin and spectinomycin have limited uses.) Resistance of Gram-negative bacilli to aminoglycosides is caused by adenylating, acetylating, or phosphorylating enzymes produced by the bacteria, which inactivate the antibiotic. The specific activities are highly variable. As a result, antibiotic susceptibility tests must be done for each aminoglycoside drug separately. Kanamycin is not effective against *Pseudomonas aeruginosa*; the other drugs are preferred whenever that infection is present or suspected. There are small differences in comparative toxicities of these aminoglycosides to the kidneys and eighth cranial nerve. In animal models netilmicin is the least toxic. It is possible that netilmicin and tobramycin are the safest, but there are conflicting reports in studies focusing on small changes in renal function rather than on frank renal failure. It is uncertain whether these small differences are clinically significant. In any case, it is advisable to monitor peak and trough serum concentrations in all patients; elevated peak and trough concentrations correlate with toxicity. With amikacin and kanamycin, desired peak concentrations are 20–35 μg/ml and trough drug concentrations are less than 10 μg/ml; for the others they are 5–10 μg/ml and less than 2 μg/ml, respectively. Patients with cystic fibrosis require larger-than-normal dosages to achieve therapeutic serum concentrations, and they excrete aminoglycosides more rapidly. **Once Daily Dosing.** Once daily dosing of 5–6 mg/kg gentamicin or tobramycin has been used in some children; peak serum concentrations are greater than those achieved with thrice daily dosing. Aminoglycosides demonstrate concentration-dependent killing of organisms, suggesting a potential benefit to higher serum concentrations achieved with once daily dosing. Regimens giving the daily dosage as a single infusion, rather than as traditional split doses every 8 hours, are safe and effective in adults and may be less toxic. Experience with once daily dosing in children is limited to date, but may become the standard after further study. In the case of nosocomial infection, the choice among aminoglycosides should be based on knowledge of local susceptibility patterns. In addition to routine monitoring of *in vitro* susceptibility testing results to detect emergence of resistant strains, the policy of switching among the drugs for routine hospital use every 1–2 years might minimize the likelihood of resistance due to selective drug pressure.

**Oral Cephalosporins** (cefaclor, cefadroxil, cefdinir, cefixime, cefpodoxime, cefprozil, ceftibuten, cefuroxime axetil, cephalexin, cephradine, and loracarbef). As a class, the oral cephalosporins have the advantages over oral penicillins of somewhat greater safety and greater palatability of the suspension formulations. (Penicillins have a bitter taste.) Cefuroxime and cefpodoxime, which are esters, are the least palatable. Cephalexin and cephradine have virtually identical properties and effectiveness and can be used interchangeably. The half-lives of cefadroxil, cefpodoxime, cefprozil, ceftibuten, and loracarbef in serum are approximately twice as long as those of the other drugs. This pharmacokinetic feature accounts for the fact that they can be given in only one or two daily doses. Cefaclor, cefdinir, cefixime, cefpodoxime, cefprozil, ceftibuten, cefuroxime, and loracarbef have the advantage of adding *Haemophilus influenzae* (including beta-lactamase–producing strains) to the spectrum.

**Parenteral Cephalosporins.** First generation cephalosporins (cefazolin, cephalothin, cephapirin, and cephradine) have been used mainly as drugs for treatment of Gram-positive infections because their Gram-negative spectrum is limited. Cefazolin is tolerated best on intramuscular injection; furthermore, it is given q8h, because of its longer half-life in serum, rather than on the q4–6h schedules used for the others. Differences in the frequencies of vein irritation among the group are minor.

The second generation cephalosporins (cefamandole, cefuroxime and cefonicid) and cephamycins (cefoxitin and cefotetan) added to the antibacterial spectrum. Cefoxitin has good activity against approximately 80% of *Bacteroides fragilis* and can be considered for use in place of metronidazole, clindamycin or chloramphenicol when that organism is implicated in disease. Cefotetan has a spectrum similar to that of cefoxitin but a longer serum half life, so it can be given q12h. Cefamandole and cefuroxime added *H. influenzae* to the spectrum of cephalosporins. However, cefamandole is somewhat unstable to the TEM1 beta-lactamase elaborated by *H. influenzae*. This characteristic, combined with its rather poor penetration into cerebrospinal fluid, resulted in cases of *Haemophilus* meningitis developing in infants treated with cefamandole. Cefuroxime is more stable to the enzyme and has better penetration into CSF (comparable to that of ampicillin). It has been used to treat meningitis due to the usual pathogens; however, reports of delayed sterilization of CSF limit its use for meningitis. Cefuroxime has utility as single drug therapy (in place of combinations such as nafcillin and chloramphenicol) for infants and young children with pneumonia, bone and joint infections, or other conditions in which Gram-positive cocci and *Haemophilus* are the usual pathogens. Because of the substantial decrease of *H. influenzae* type b following adoption of routine immunization of infants against that organism, this advantage of cefuroxime is less important than in the past, although cefuroxime does retain significant activity against penicillin nonsusceptible strains of pneumococcus.

Third generation cephalosporins (cefoperazone, cefotaxime, ceftriaxone, ceftizoxime, and ceftazidime) all have enhanced potency against many Gram-negative bacilli, usually including aminoglycoside-resistant organisms. They are inactive against enterococci and *Listeria* and have variable activity against *Pseudomonas* and

*Bacteroides*. Cefotaxime and ceftriaxone have been used successfully to treat meningitis caused by the usual pathogens. Limited experience with ceftazidime and ceftizoxime suggests that they too are effective for meningitis. These drugs have greatest usefulness for treating Gram-negative bacillary infections when aminoglycosides are contraindicated or when the organisms are resistant to customarily used drugs. Because cefoperazone and ceftriaxone are excreted to a large extent via the liver, they can be used with little dosage adjustment in patients with renal failure. Ceftazidime has the unique property of activity against *P. aeruginosa* that is comparable to that of the aminoglycosides. Ceftriaxone has a serum half-life of 4–7 hours and can be given once a day.

Cefepime, a fourth generation cephalosporin approved for use in children, exhibits both the antipseudomonal activity of ceftazidime and the Gram-positive activity of second generation cephalosporins. Limited published experience suggests efficacy in the therapy of pediatric meningitis caused by the usual pathogens, but cefepime is not FDA-approved for that indication in the United States.

**Penicillinase-Resistant Penicillins** (cloxacillin, dicloxacillin, methicillin, nafcillin, and oxacillin). Nafcillin differs pharmacologically from the others in being excreted primarily by the liver rather than by the kidneys. This may be the reason for its lack of nephrotoxicity. Nephrotoxicity or hemorrhagic cystitis occurs in 5% of children treated with methicillin. For this reason nafcillin is preferred over methicillin for parenteral use with two exceptions: in neonates and in patients with hepatic disease. Nafcillin pharmacokinetics in the newborn are erratic, especially in jaundiced babies; furthermore, methicillin nephrotoxicity is rare in the neonate. Nafcillin pharmacokinetics are also erratic in persons with liver disease. For oral use, cloxacillin, oxacillin, and dicloxacillin are essentially equivalent, but the latter has the greatest antistaphylococcal activity *in vitro*.

**Antipseudomonal Beta-Lactams** (mezlocillin, piperacillin, ticarcillin, ticarcillin-clavulanate, piperacillin-tazobactam, aztreonam, ceftazidime, cefepime, meropenem, and imipenem). Ceftazidime, cefepime, meropenem, and imipenem have the most active *in vitro* against *Pseudomonas*. Mezlocillin does not affect platelet adhesiveness significantly, but the other penicillins do; this could be an advantage in patients who have another risk factor for bleeding. In general, *Pseudomonas* strains resistant to ticarcillin are resistant to the newer drugs except for meropenem and imipenem. These drugs should be used along with an aminoglycoside for treating *Pseudomonas* infections in compromised hosts for synergistic effect. The combination of penicillin/beta-lactamase inhibitor (ticarcillin/clavulanate, Timentin®; and piperacillin/tazobactam, Zosyn®) have little added effect on activity against *Pseudomonas* but do extend the spectrum to many beta-lactamase–positive bacteria.

**Aminopenicillins** (amoxicillin, amoxicillin-clavulanate, ampicillin, ampicillin-sulbactam, bacampicillin). Because bacampicillin is rapidly and completely converted in the body to ampicillin, it is an indirect means of administering ampicillin.

Bacampicillin is the most efficiently absorbed, and peak blood concentrations are greater than after the same dosage of amoxicillin or ampicillin. Ampicillin is more likely than the others to cause diarrhea and to disturb colonic coliform flora and cause overgrowth of *Candida*. Augmentin® is a combination of amoxicillin and clavulanate for oral use that permits amoxicillin to be active against many beta-lactamase–producing bacteria. Sulbactam, another beta-lactamase inhibitor, is combined with ampicillin in the parenteral formulation, Unasyn®. Clinical experience is too limited to assess its role in pediatric patients.

**Carbapenems.** Meropenem and imipenem are carbapenems with a broader spectrum of activity than any other beta-lactams currently available. Both meropenem and imipenem are approved by the FDA for use in children. At present they are recommended for treatment of infections caused by bacteria resistant to most other drugs, or mixed infections involving both aerobes and anaerobes. Imipenem has CNS toxicity, especially in patients with meningitis, but this has not been a problem to date with meropenem. They are active against coliform bacilli and *P. aeruginosa* (including most third generation cephalosporin–resistant strains) as well as against anaerobes, including *B. fragilis*.

**Macrolides.** Erythromycin is the prototype of a class called macrolide antibiotics. Almost 30 macrolides have been produced, but only four are commercially available in the United States: erythromycin, azithromycin, clarithromycin, and dirithromycin. (Azithromycin is actually an azalide compound structurally similar to macrolides.) As a class, these drugs achieve greater concentrations in tissues than in serum. (Tissue concentrations are markedly greater with azithromycin and clarithromycin than with erythromycin.) As a result, measuring serum concentrations is not clinically useful. Erythromycin has poor gastrointestinal tolerance in many patients. This is less of a problem with the newer drugs. Erythromycin suspensions are ester formulations and must be hydrolyzed to the active base compound. The estolate form results in greater serum and tissue concentrations of erythromycin than do the other esters. Macrolides have the broadest range of antimicrobial activity of all classes of antibiotics approved for use in children. This is especially true of azithromycin and clarithromycin, which are demonstrating clinical utility greater than that of erythromycin in *H. influenzae*, chlamydial, and mycobacterial infections.

# III. ANTIBIOTIC THERAPY FOR NEWBORNS

## A. RECOMMENDED THERAPY FOR SELECTED CONDITIONS

NOTE: To avoid repetition, the recommended dosages and intervals of administration of antibiotics indicated with an asterisk in most of the following conditions are given in the Table on pages 16 and 17.

| Condition | Therapy | Comment |
|---|---|---|
| **Congenital syphilis** | Aqueous penicillin G 50,000 U/kg q12h (day of life 1–7), q8h (> 7 days) IV OR procaine penicillin G 50,000 U/kg IM once daily; × 10–14 days; Optional alternative for asymptomatic infant or when infant's nontreponemal test is negative: benzathine penicillin G 50,000 U/kg IM, single dose | Obtain follow-up serology at 3, 6, and 12 mos until nontreponemal test nonreactive or decreased fourfold |
| **Congenital toxoplasmosis** | Sulfadiazine 100 mg/kg/day PO div q6–12h AND pyrimethamine 2 mg/kg PO daily × 2 (loading dose), then 1 mg/kg PO once daily for 6 wks, then 3 times weekly up to 1 yr; Alternative: pyrimethamine (as above) AND clindamycin* | Supplemental folinic acid 5–10 mg 3 times weekly; Steroids if chorioretinitis or CSF protein > 1 g/dl |
| **Herpes simplex infection** | Acyclovir 60 mg/kg/day as 1–2 hr IV infusion div q8h × 21 days for CNS and disseminated disease, or × 14 days for other types; PLUS trifluridine ophthalmic solution topically q2h for conjunctivitis (max 9 times/day) | Larger dosages of acyclovir and more days of Rx than previously recommended may be beneficial |
| **Human immunodeficiency virus infection** | Term baby: zidovudine 8 mg/kg/day PO div q6h OR 6 mg/kg/day IV div q6h; Preterm baby (≤ 34 wks): 3 mg/kg/day IV, PO div q12h × 2 wks, then 6 mg/kg/day IV, PO div q8h × 6 wks | For infants born to HIV-positive mothers; Single dose nivirapine 2 mg/kg PO being tested |

| | | |
|---|---|---|
| **Tetanus neonatorum** | Penicillin G* IV × 10 days | Antitoxin and sedation; Do not use IM injections |
| **Parotitis, suppurative** | Oxacillin* IV <u>AND</u> aminoglycoside IV, IM × 10 days | Usually staphylococcal but occasionally coliform |
| **Conjunctivitis** | | |
| - Chlamydial | Erythromycin* estolate or ethylsuccinate PO × 10–14 days <u>OR</u> topical erythromycin, tetracycline, or sulfacetamide ointment q.i.d. | Erythro PO preferable to topical therapy because NP carrier state eradicated; Treat mother and her sexual partner |
| - Gonococcal | Ceftriaxone 25–50 mg/kg (max 125 mg) IV, IM <u>OR</u> cefotaxime 100 mg/kg IV, IM as single dose; (More than 1 day of therapy may be used for severe cases) | Saline irrigation of eyes; Treat mother and her sexual partner; Evaluate for chlamydial infection |
| - *Staphylococcus aureus* | Oxacillin* IM, IV × 7–10 days (topical therapy only for mild cases) | Additionally: neomycin ophthalmic drops or ointment |
| - *Pseudomonas aeruginosa* | Ticarcillin* or mezlocillin* IV, IM <u>AND</u> aminoglycoside* IM, IV × 7–10 days (Alternative: ceftazidime*) | Polymyxin B ophthalmic drops or ointment; Subtenon or subconjunctival antibiotics in some cases |
| **Gastrointestinal infections** | | |
| - *Salmonella* | Cefotaxime* IV, IM × 7–10 days if suspected sepsis or focal infection | Observe for focal complications (meningitis, arthritis, etc.) |
| - Necrotizing enterocolitis or peritonitis secondary to bowel rupture | Ticarcillin* IV, IM <u>AND</u> aminoglycoside* IM, IV × 10 days or longer; Cefotaxime* suitable alternative to aminoglycoside; Vancomycin* IV if *Staphylococcus epidermidis* or methicillin-resistant *Staphylococcus* cultured; Common alternative: vancomycin* + aminoglycoside* ± clindamycin* | Bacteremia in 30–50% of cases; After 2–3 days of age, *Bacteroides* common in gut; Clindamycin* or metronidazole* for ticarcillin-resistant *B. fragilis* |

*See pages 16–17 for dosage

| Condition | Therapy | Comment |
|---|---|---|
| **Sepsis and meningitis** | NOTE: Duration of therapy: 7–10 days for sepsis without a focus; 21 days minimum for Gram-negative meningitis; 14 days minimum for group B streptococcal meningitis | |
| - Initial therapy, organism unknown | Ampicillin* IV AND cefotaxime* IV, IM | Ampicillin* AND aminoglycoside* is a suitable alternative |
| - *Bacteroides fragilis* spp. *fragilis* | Metronidazole,* clindamycin,* mezlocillin,* or ticarcillin* IV, IM | Metronidazole preferred for CNS infection |
| - Coliform bacteria | Cefotaxime* IV, IM; Lumbar intrathecal or intraventricular injections of aminoglycoside are not beneficial in usual case | Aminoglycoside* is suitable alternative; (?) Meropenem for aminoglycoside/ cephalosporin-resistant organism |
| - Group A | Penicillin G* IV | |
| - Group B streptococcus | Ampicillin* or penicillin G* IV AND gentamicin* IV IM (Discontinue gentamicin when sterilization achieved) | Synergy may be advantage especially against penicillin-tolerant strains |
| - Enterococcal sp. | Ampicillin* IV, IM AND aminoglycoside* IV, IM | Vancomycin* for ampicillin-resistant organism |
| - Gonococcal | Ceftriaxone 25–50 mg/kg IV, IM once daily OR cefotaxime 100 mg/kg/day IV, IM div q12h | Duration of therapy uncertain (? 5 days) |
| - *Listeria monocytogenes* | Ampicillin* IV, IM AND aminoglycoside* IV, IM | Aminoglycosides synergistic *in vitro* with ampicillin |
| - *Staphylococcus epidermidis* | Vancomycin* IV | Usually methicillin-resistant |
| - *Staphylococcus aureus* | Oxacillin* IV, IM; Vancomycin* IV for methicillin-resistant *Staphylococcus* | Nafcillin may be preferable for meningitis |

| | | |
|---|---|---|
| - *Pseudomonas aeruginosa* | Mezlocillin* or ticarcillin* IV, IM <u>AND</u> aminoglycoside* IV, IM | Ceftazidime* and aminoglycoside* is a suitable alternative |
| **Osteomyelitis, suppurative arthritis** | | Surgical drainage of pus; Physical therapy |
| - Gonococcal arthritis and tenosynovitis | Ceftriaxone* 25–50 mg/kg IV, IM once daily × 7–10 days | |
| - *Staphylococcus aureus* | Oxacillin* IV, IM × 21 days minimum; Vancomycin* IV for methicillin-resistant *Staphylococcus* | Change to penicillin G if organism susceptible |
| - Coliform bacteria | Cefotaxime* <u>OR</u> aminoglycoside* IV, IM × 21 days minimum | Cephalosporins better than aminoglycosides for deep tissue infection |
| - Group B streptococcus | (See Group B streptococcal meningitis) | |
| - Unknown | Oxacillin* IV, IM <u>AND</u> cefotaxime* IV, IM × 21 days minimum | |
| **Otitis media** | Few controlled treatment trials in newborns; Suggest using initial therapy as for older infants (see page 24); If no response, obtain middle ear fluid for culture | Augmentin may have advantage because of activity against coliforms and *Staphylococcus* (10–20% of cases) |
| - Coliform bacteria | Augmentin 30–40 mg/kg/day PO div q8–12h × 10 days | Cefotaxime* if parenteral therapy needed |
| - *Staphylococcus aureus* | Cloxacillin or cephalexin 50 mg/kg/day PO div q6–8h × 10 days | Oxacillin* if unable to treat PO |
| - Streptococcus | Penicillin V 30 mg/kg/day PO div q8h × 10 days | May be given IV |
| - *Haemophilus* | Augmentin 30–40 mg/kg/day PO div q8–12h OR amoxicillin 30–40 mg/kg/day PO div q8–12 if susceptible | |

*See pages 16–17 for dosage

| Condition | Therapy | Comment |
|---|---|---|
| **Pulmonary infections** | | |
| - *Staphylococcus aureus* | Oxacillin* IV, IM × 21 days minimum; Vancomycin* IV for methicillin-resistant *Staphylococcus* | Closed tube drainage of empyema |
| - *Pseudomonas aeruginosa* | Mezlocillin* or ticarcillin* IV, IM AND aminoglycoside* IV, IM × 14 days or longer | Ceftazidime* is a suitable alternative |
| - Group B streptococcus | Penicillin G* IV OR ampicillin* IV, IM × 10–14 days | Radiograph often mimics hyaline membrane disease |
| - *Chlamydia trachomatis* | Erythromycin* PO × 14–21 days | Ampicillin, amoxicillin, or sulfa drugs may be effective |
| - Aspiration pneumonia | Oxacillin* IV, IM AND aminoglycoside* IV, IM × 7–10 days | Mild aspiration episodes do not require antibiotic therapy |
| - *Ureaplasma urealyticum* | Clarithromycin 30 mg/kg/day PO div q12h × 10 days; (? doxycycline for CNS infection) | Pathogenic role of *Ureaplasma* uncertain |
| - Pertussis | Erythromycin* × 14 days OR ampicillin* IV, IM if PO meds not retained | Usually acquired from parent or other adult in household |
| **Skin and soft tissues** | | |
| - Impetigo neonatorum | Cleansing alone OR oxacillin* IV, IM OR cephalexin 50 mg/kg/day PO div q6–8h OR mupirocin topically; × 5 days | No antibiotic for superficial impetigo; Chlorhexidine baths; Break lesions with alcohol swab |
| - Erysipelas (and other Group A streptococcal infections) | Penicillin G* IV × 5–7 days | Group B streptococcus may produce similar cellulitis or nodular lesions |
| - Breast abscess | Oxacillin* IV, IM ( 5–7 days; aminoglycoside* OR cefotaxime* if Gram-negative rods seen in pus | Gram stain of expressed pus/colostrum or I&D material (Avoid damage to breast tissue) |

| | | |
|---|---|---|
| - *Staphylococcus* | Oxacillin* IV, IM × 5–7 days; Vancomycin* for methicillin-resistant *Staphylococcus* | Value of systemic antibiotics over surgical drainage alone not established |
| - Group B streptococcus | Penicillin G* IV OR ampicillin* IV, IM; × 5–7 days | Usually no pus formed |
| - Omphalitis and funisitis | | |
| Group A or B streptococci | Penicillin G* IV × 5–7 days OR (for Group A strep) benzathine penicillin G 50,000 U/kg IM × 1 dose PLUS topical "triple dye" or bacitracin ointment | Group A strep usually causes "wet cord" without pus and with minimal erythema |
| *Staphylococcus aureus* | Oxacillin* IV, IM × 5 days or longer | Observe for bacteremia and other focus of infection |
| Necrotizing funisitis | Oxacillin* IV, IM AND aminoglycoside* IV, IM | Unknown etiology but secondary infection may occur |
| Clostridial | Clindamycin* AND cefotaxime* × 10 days or longer | Crepitance and rapidly spreading cellulitis around umbilicus |
| **Urinary tract infection** | Initial empiric therapy usually with ampicillin* and gentamicin* pending culture and susceptibility test results | Investigate for abnormalities of urinary tract |
| - Coliform bacteria | Gentamicin* IV, IM OR cefotaxime* IV, IM × 10 days | Ampicillin used for susceptible organisms |
| - *Pseudomonas aeruginosa* | Mezlocillin* or ticarcillin* IV, IM AND aminoglycoside* IV, IM × 10 days | Ceftazidime* is a suitable alternative |
| - *Enterococcus* | Ampicillin* IV, IM AND aminoglycoside* × 10 days | Vancomycin if ampicillin-resistant |

*See pages 16–17 for dosage

## B. USE OF ANTIMICROBIALS DURING PREGNANCY OR BREASTFEEDING

A number of factors determine the degree of transfer of antibiotics across the placenta: lipid solubility, degree of ionization, molecular weight, protein binding, placental maturation, and placental and fetal blood flow. During the latter part of pregnancy maternal serum concentrations of most antibiotics decrease because of the increased volume of distribution. Fetal serum concentrations of the following drugs are equal to, or only slightly less than, those in the mother: penicillin G, amoxicillin, ampicillin, carbenicillin, methicillin, sulfonamides, trimethoprim, tetracyclines, nitrofurantoin, and chloramphenicol. The aminoglycoside concentrations in fetal serum are 20–50% of those in maternal serum. Cephalosporins, nafcillin, oxacillin, clindamycin, and colistimethate penetrate poorly (10–15%) and fetal concentrations of erythromycin and dicloxacillin are less than 10% of those in the mother.

Some drugs can cause harm to the pregnant woman or fetus. Drugs that are contraindicated are: ribavirin, amantadine, cinoxacin, ciprofloxacin, norfloxacin, erythromycin estolate, griseofulvin, nalidixic acid, tetracyclines, emetine, lindane, and primaquine. Drugs that are considered safe are: penicillins, aztreonam, cephalosporins, erythromycin base, methenamine mandelate, spectinomycin, nystatin, chloroquine, niclosamide, paromomycin, permethrin, praziquantel, pyrantel pamoate, and pyrethrins. Drugs not listed should be used with caution for firm clinical indications (Med Lett 1987;29:61).

Concentrations of antibiotics in human breast milk are not well studied. Isoniazid, metronidazole, trimethoprim, and sulfonamides occur in equal concentrations in maternal serum and milk. Tetracyclines, chloramphenicol, and erythromycin are found in breast milk in concentrations 50–75% of those in serum. Breast milk concentrations of penicillin G and V, aminoglycosides, nalidixic acid, oxacillin, novobiocin, various cephalosporins, and nitrofurantoin have been reported to be less than 25% of the maternal serum concentrations. Because these are microgram amounts, they would not be ingested by the infant in therapeutic amounts.

For example, if an infant took 110 cc/kg body weight of breast milk containing 10 µg/ml isoniazid in a day, this would amount to a "dose" of 1.1 mg/kg/day. The same infant ingesting milk containing 10 mg/dl of sulfonamide would receive 11 mg/kg/day. On the other hand, with a penicillin V concentration of 0.1 µg/ml in breast milk, the amount of penicillin taken in by the infant would be only 0.011 mg/kg/day.

Antibiotics are usually compatible with breastfeeding, but the AAP Committee on Drugs warns about the possibility of inducing hemolysis in babies with G-6-PD deficiency by nalidixic acid, nitrofurantoin, or sulfa drugs (Transfer of drugs and other chemicals into human milk. Pediatrics 1994;93:137).

## C. TABLE OF ANTIBIOTIC DOSAGES FOR NEONATES

| Antibiotics | Routes of Administration | Dosages (mg/kg/day) and Intervals of Administration | | | | |
|---|---|---|---|---|---|---|
| | | Body Weight < 2000 g | | Body Weight > 2000 g | | |
| | | 0–7 days old | 8–28 days old | 0–7 days old | 8–28 days old | > 28 days old |
| Ampicillin | IV, IM | 100 div q12h | 150 div q8h | 150 div q8h | 200 div q6h | 200 div q6h |
| Aztreonam | IV | 60 div q12h | 90 div q8h | 90 div q8h | 120 div q6h | 120 div q6h |
| Cefazolin | IV, IM | 40 div q12h | 40 div q12h | 40 div q12h | 60 div q8h | 60 div q8h |
| Cefotaxime | IV, IM | 100 div q12h | 150 div q8h | 100 div q12h | 150 div q8h | 200 div q6h |
| Ceftazidime | IV, IM | 100 div q12h | 150 div q8h | 100 div q12h | 150 div q8h | 150 div q8h |
| Ceftriaxone | IV, IM | 50 once daily | 50 once daily | 50 once daily | 75 once daily | 100 once daily |
| Cefuroxime | IV, IM | 100 div q12h | 150 div q8h | 150 div q8h | 150 div q8h | 150 div q8h |
| Clindamycin | IV, IM, PO | 10 div q12h | 15 div q8h | 15 div q8h | 20 div q6h | 30 div q6h |
| Erythromycin | IV, PO | 20 div q12h | 30 div q8h | 20 div q12h | 40 div q8h | 40 div q6h |
| Metronidazole | IV, PO | 7.5 div q24h | 15 div q12h | 15 div q12h | 30 div q12h | 30 div q6h |
| Mezlocillin | IV, IM | 150 div q12h | 225 div q8h | 150 div q12h | 225 div q8h | 300 div q6h |
| Nafcillin, oxacillin | IV | 50 div q12h | 75 div q8h | 75 div q8h | 150 div q6h | 150 div q6h |
| Penicillin G | IV | 100,000 U div q12h | 225,000 U div q8h | 150,000 U div q8h | 200,000 U div q6h | 200,000 U div q6h |
| Procaine Penicillin G | IM | 50,000 U q24h | 50,000 U q24h | 50,000 U q24h | 50,000 U q24h | 50,000 U q24h |
| Ticarcillin | IV, IM | 150 div q12h | 225 div q8h | 225 div q8h | 300 div q6h | 300 div q6h |

## D. DRUGS FOR NEONATES DOSED ACCORDING ONLY TO AGE

| Drug | Routes of Administration | Dosage (mg/kg/dose) by Gestational Age Plus Weeks of Life | | | |
|---|---|---|---|---|---|
| | | ≤ 26 Wks | 27–34 Wks | 35–42 Wks | ≥ 43 Wks |
| Acyclovir | IV | 20 q12h | 20 q12h | 20 q8h | 20 q8h |
| Amikacin[a] | IV, IM | 7.5 q24h | 7.5 q18h | 10 q12h | 10 q8h |
| Gentamicin[b] | IV, IM | 2.5 q24h | 2.5 q18h | 2.5 q12h[d] | 2.5 q8h[d] |
| Tobramycin[b] | IV, IM | 2.5 q24h | 2.5 q18h | 2.5 q12h | 2.5 q8h |
| Vancomycin[c] | IV | 15 q24h | 15 q18h[e] | 15 q12h[e] | 15 q8h[e] |

[a]Desired serum concentrations: 20–30 μg/ml (peak), < 10 μg/ml (trough)
[b]Desired serum concentrations: 5–10 mg/ml (peak), < 2.5 mg/ml (trough)
[c]Desired serum concentrations: 20–40 mg/ml (peak), < 10 mg/ml (trough)
[d]Once daily dosing regimen (4 mg/kg) is used by some neonatologists.
[e]At 28 days of life (4 weeks) vancomycin is dosed at 20 mg/kg/dose. The interval remains the same.

(Table prepared by Pablo J. Sánchez, MD)

# IV. ANTIMICROBIAL THERAPY ACCORDING TO CLINICAL SYNDROMES

NOTES:
1. This tabulation should be considered a rough guideline for the "usual" patient. Deviations should be made according to physiologic peculiarities of the patient. Dosages recommended are for patients with normal or nearly normal hydration, renal function, and hepatic function. See Section XII for information on patients with impaired renal function and Section XV for dosages based on square meters of body surface area.
2. Duration of treatment should be individualized. The periods recommended are based on common practice and general experience. Critical evaluations of duration of therapy have been carried out in very few diseases.
3. Diseases are arranged by body systems. Consult the index for the alphabetized listing of diseases and Section VII for the alphabetized listing of etiologic agents and for uncommon agents not included in this section.

| Clinical Diagnosis | Therapy | Comments |
|---|---|---|
| **A. SKIN AND SOFT TISSUE INFECTIONS** | | |
| NOTE: Erythromycin for penicillin-allergic patients. | | |
| **Streptococcal cellulitis** (erysipelas) | Penicillin G 50,000–100,000 U/kg/day, IV div q4–6h initially then penicillin V 50 mg (80,000 U)/kg/day PO div q6–8h OR amoxicillin 50/kg/day div q8h × 10 days | These dosages may be unnecessarily large but there is little clinical experience with smaller dosages |
| **Lymphangitis, lymphadenitis, blistering dactylitis** (streptococcal) | Penicillin V 25–50 mg (40,000–80,000 U)/kg/day PO div q6–8h OR erythromycin 40–50 mg/kg/day PO div q8–12h; × 10 days | For severe disease, penicillin IV (as above) |
| **Impetigo** | Mupirocin topically to lesions t.i.d.; OR (for extensive lesions) erythromycin (as above) or cephalexin 50–75 mg/kg/day PO div q8h | Bathe daily; Usually mixed streptococcal and staphylococcal infection |
| **Bullous impetigo, staphylococcal scarlet fever** | Cephalexin 50–75 mg/kg/day PO div q8h; OR cloxacillin 50 mg/kg/day PO div q6h; × 5–7 days | Other antistaphylococcal drugs can be used |

| | | |
|---|---|---|
| **Scalded skin syndrome** | Oxacillin 150 mg/kg/day IV div q6h or cefazolin 100 mg/kg/day IV div q8h initially; then cloxacillin OR cephalexin (as above); × 5–7 days | Burow's or Zephiran compresses for intertriginous areas |
| **Pyoderma, abscesses, cervical adenitis, Ludwig's angina** (streptococcal, staphylococcal) | Cephalexin 50–75 mg/kg/day PO div q8h; OR cloxacillin (as above); × 5–10 days | I&D when indicated; Oxacillin IV for serious infections |
| **Necrotizing fasciitis** (streptococcal, staphylococcal) | Oxacillin 150 mg/kg/day IV div q6h or cefazolin 100 mg/kg/day IV div q8h × 10 days (Alternative: meropenem or imipenem if Gram-negative or mixed aerobic/anaerobic infection suspected) | Aggressive, emergent debridement; For streptococcal infection with toxic shock, consider a combination of penicillin and clindamycin; Consider IVIG to bind toxin |
| **Cellulitis of unknown etiology** (Usually *S. aureus* or *Streptococcus pyogenes*) | Oxacillin 150 mg/kg/day IV div q6h or cefazolin 100 mg/kg/day IV div q8h initially; Then cephalexin 50–75 mg/kg/day PO div q8h OR cloxacillin 50 mg/kg/day PO div q6h × 7–10 days | For unimmunized infants, consider *H. influenzae*, type b for buccal or periorbital cellulitis (q.v.) |
| **Buccal cellulitis** (*H. influenzae*, type b) | Cefotaxime 100–150 mg/kg/day IV div q6h OR ceftriaxone 50 mg/kg/day IV, IM q24h OR chloramphenicol 50–75 mg/kg/day IV div q6h; × 5–7 days | R/O meningitis (larger dosages may be needed) |
| **Suppurative myositis** (staphylococcal) (synonyms: tropical myositis, pyomyositis) | Oxacillin 150 mg/kg/day IV div q6h OR cefazolin 100 mg/kg/day IV div q8h × 7–10 days; Alternatives: other antistaphylococcal beta-lactams, vancomycin | Surgical drainage or excision when needed |
| **Gas gangrene** (clostridial) | Penicillin G 250,000 U/kg/day IV div q4h × 10 days; For penicillin allergy, consider clindamycin or meropenem | Aggressive, extensive debridement; Antitoxin was of doubtful efficacy and is no longer available |

| Clinical Diagnosis | Therapy | Comments |
|---|---|---|
| **Nontuberculous (atypical) mycobacterial adenitis** | Total surgical excision, if possible, is usually curative and antimicrobial therapy is not necessary in non-immunocompromised patient | If surgical excision not possible, azithromycin or clarithromycin therapy if organisms susceptible |
| **Tuberculous adenitis** | As for pulmonary tuberculosis (See page 31) | Surgical excision usually not indicated |
| **Animal and human bites** | | |
| - *Pasteurella multocida* (animal), *Eikenella corrodens* (human), *Staphylococcus* sp. and *Streptococcus* sp. | Augmentin® 20–40 mg/kg/day PO div q8h × 5–7 days; For hospitalized patients use Timentin®, 200 mg ticarcillin component/kg/day div q6h OR ampicillin and clindamycin | Human bites often mixed aerobes and anaerobes; Consider rabies prophylaxis for animal bites; Tetanus prophylaxis |
| - Rat-bite fever (*Streptobacillus moniliformis*, *Spirillum minus*) | Penicillin G 50–100,000 U/kg/day IV div q6h × 7–10 days; For endocarditis, × 4–6 wks | |

B. SKELETAL INFECTIONS

See Section XI for discussion of Oral Antibiotic Therapy

| Clinical Diagnosis | Therapy | Comments |
|---|---|---|
| **Suppurative arthritis** | | Needle aspiration or surgical drainage; Physiotherapy |
| - Newborns | See Section III | |
| - Infants (*Haemophilus,* streptococci, *Staphylococcus*) | Cefuroxime or cefotaxime 100–150 mg/kg/day IV, IM div q8h OR (for streptococcus) penicillin G 100,000 U/kg/day IV div q4–6h × 14 days or longer OR (for *Staphylococcus*) oxacillin 150 mg/kg/day IV div q6h or cefazolin 100 mg/kg/day IV div q8h × 21 days or longer | *Haemophilus* unlikely in immunized populations |

| | | |
|---|---|---|
| - Children (*Staphylococcus*, streptococci) | Oxacillin 150 mg/kg/day IV div q6h <u>OR</u> cefazolin 100 mg/kg/day IV div q8h × 3 wks or longer; Alternatives: other beta-lactams, clindamycin; vancomycin for methicillin-resistant staphylococci | Ceftriaxone or cefotaxime for penicillin-resistant pneumococcus |
| - Gonococcal arthritis or tenosynovitis | Ceftriaxone 50 mg/kg once daily IV, IM <u>OR</u> (if susceptible) penicillin G 100,000 U/kg/day IV div q6h; × 7–10 days | 3–5 days therapy adequate in adults but not tested in children |
| - Other bacteria | See Section V for preferred antibiotics | |
| **Osteomyelitis or osteochondritis** | | Surgery; Immobilization |
| - Newborn | See Section III | |
| - Acute, initial therapy (usually *Staphylococcus*, streptococci) | Oxacillin 150 mg/kg/day IV, div q6h <u>OR</u> cefazolin 100 mg/kg/day IV div q8h; × 3 wks or longer. Alternatives: other beta-lactams, clindamycin | Consider *Haemophilus* if unimmunized; In children add ceftazidime to nafcillin if Gram-negative rods in pus, pending culture and susceptibility results |
| - Acute, other organisms | See Section V for preferred antibiotics | |
| - *Pseudomonas aeruginosa* | Ceftazidime 150 mg/kg/day IV, IM div q8h <u>OR</u> mezlocillin or ticarcillin 200–300 mg/kg/day IV div q6h <u>AND</u> (compromised host) gentamicin 6–7.5 mg/kg/day IM, IV or amikacin 15–20 mg/kg/day IM, IV div q8h; × 10 days | If thorough surgical debridement not done, longer therapy required and may not be curative |
| - Chronic (staphylococcal) | Dicloxacillin 75–100 mg/kg/day PO div q6h <u>OR</u> cephalexin 100–150 mg/kg/day PO div q6h; × 6–12 mos | Surgery; Monitor serum for bactericidal titer or antibiotic concentration (See Section XI for details) |

| Clinical Diagnosis | Therapy | Comments |
|---|---|---|
| C. EYE INFECTIONS | | |
| **Hordeolum (sty) or chalazion** | None (Topical antibiotic not necessary) | Warm compresses; I&D when necessary |
| **Acute conjunctivitis** | Polymyxin B-bacitracin or sulfacetamide ophthalmic drops q2h or ointment q4–6h | See page 9 for chlamydial, gonococcal, pseudomonal infection |
| **Herpetic conjunctivitis** | Trifluridine solution 1 drop q2–3h while awake × 7–14 days; OR vidarabine ointment topically q3h until 1 wk after healing | Consider steroids if keratitis present (Refer to ophthalmologist) |
| **Periorbital cellulitis** (Preseptal infection) | | |
| - Associated with periorbital skin lesion (streptococcal, staphylococcal) | Oxacillin 150 mg/kg/day IV div q6h OR cefazolin 100 mg/kg/day IV div q8h; × 7–10 days | Oral antistaphylococcal antibiotic for less severe infection |
| - Associated with sinusitis | Cefuroxime or cefotaxime 100–150 mg/kg/day IV, IM div q8h; × 5–7 days | Sinusitis may cause noninflammatory periorbital edema. Follow with oral antibiotic (See page 25) |
| - Idiopathic (pneumococcal or *H. influenzae*, type b) | Cefuroxime or cefotaxime 100–150 mg/kg/day IV, IM div q8h OR chloramphenicol 50–75 mg/kg/day IV div q6h; × 7–10 days | R/O meningitis; LARGER DOSAGES MAY BE NEEDED; Vancomycin for penicillin-resistant pneumococcal meningitis |
| **Orbital cellulitis** (Postseptal infection) | Oxacillin 150 mg/kg/day IV div q6h OR cefazolin 100 mg/kg/day IV div q8h AND cefotaxime 150 mg/kg/day div q8h; × 10–14 days | Usually staphylococcal or Gram-negative bacilli; Surgical drainage of pus |

| | | |
|---|---|---|
| Dacryocystitis | No antibiotic usually; When needed, based on Gram's stain and culture of pus | Warm compresses; May require surgical probing of nasolacrimal duct |
| **Endophthalmitis** | <u>NOTE</u>: Subconjunctival/subtenon antibiotic often needed; Steroids commonly used; May require an anterior chamber or vitreous tap for microbiological diagnosis | |
| - Staphylococcal | Oxacillin 150 mg/kg/day IV div q6h <u>OR</u> cefazolin 100 mg/kg/day IV div q8h; × 10–14 days; Alternatives: other beta-lactams or vancomycin | Penicillin for susceptible organisms |
| - Pneumococcal, meningococcal | Penicillin G 250,000 U/kg/day IV div q4h × 10–14 days (vancomycin for penicillin-resistant pneumococci) | R/O meningitis |
| - Gonococcal | Ceftriaxone 50 mg/kg once daily IV, IM × 7 days or longer | |
| - *Pseudomonas* | Mezlocillin or ticarcillin 200–300 mg/kg/day IV div q4–6h <u>AND</u> gentamicin 6–7.5 mg/kg/day IM, IV or amikacin 15–20 mg/kg/day IM, IV div q8h × 10–14 days | Piperacillin or ceftazidime are alternatives |
| **Retinitis** | | |
| - Cytomegalovirus | Ganciclovir <u>OR</u> foscarnet (See Section VIII for dosage) | |

| Clinical Diagnosis | Therapy | Comments |
|---|---|---|
| D. EAR AND SINUS INFECTIONS | | |
| **External otitis, bacterial** | Optimal therapy unknown; cleaning canal of detritus important; Antibiotic or antibiotic-steroid drops (e.g., Cortisporin suspension or fluoroquinolone solution) | Wick moistened with Burow's solution used for marked swelling of canal; For "swimmer's ear," VoSol to canal after water exposure |
| **External otitis, fungal** (otomycosis) | Topical ½ alcohol-½ vinegar solution OR 25% M-cresyl acetate (Cresylate) t.i.d. | Usually *Aspergillus*; Debride canal |
| **Furuncle of external canal** | Cephalexin 50–75 mg/kg/day PO div q8h OR cloxacillin 50 mg/kg/day PO div q6–8h | I&D; Antibiotic not necessary unless cellulitis |
| **Bullous myringitis** | Antibiotics, as for otitis media with effusion (See the following entry) | Current concept is that this is simply one manifestation of acute otitis media |
| **Otitis media, acute** | | |
| - Newborns | See Section III | |
| - Infants and children (pneumococcus, *Haemophilus*, *Moraxella* most common) | Usual therapy: amoxicillin 80–90 mg/kg/day PO div q8h<br>For failures or recurrences: amoxicillin-clavulanate 80–90 mg of amoxicillin component/kg/day PO div q8h OR cefuroxime axetil 30 mg/kg/day PO div q12h OR ceftriaxone 50 mg/kg/day IM q24h; × 1–3 doses<br>Other approved drugs (See Section VIII for dosages): azithromycin, cefaclor, cefdinir, cefixime, cefpodoxime, cefprozil, ceftibuten, clarithromycin, erythromycin-sulfisoxazole, loracarbef, trimethoprim-sulfamethoxazole | Recommendations based on CDC Working Group report (Pediatr Infect Dis J, January 1999;18:1–9.); Gram's stain and cultures of pus, if available; If compromised host, suspect unusual infection (Tympanocentesis for culture may be necessary) |

**A Note on Acute Otitis Media with Effusion:** Several antibiotic regimens are effective for acute otitis media (AOM). Customarily, amoxicillin is used initially and other drugs are given for amoxicillin failures or relapses. The physician should consider advantages and disadvantages regarding antibacterial spectrum, palatability of suspensions, and cost. TMP/SMX is not effective for group A streptococcal infection. When prophylaxis is indicated, use amoxicillin or sulfa drug in one-half the therapeutic dose once or twice daily. How penicillin resistance in pneumococci affects empiric therapy is an unresolved issue.

| | | |
|---|---|---|
| **Mastoiditis, acute** (*Pneumococcus*, *Staphylococcus*, Group A streptococcus; *Haemophilus* rare) | Oxacillin 150 mg/kg/day IV div q6h OR cefazolin 100 mg/kg/day IV div q8h OR cefuroxime 100–150 mg/kg/day IV, IM div q8h × 10 days; Alternatives: other beta-lactams or vancomycin for penicillin-resistant pneumococci | R/O meningitis; Surgery as needed; Change to oral therapy after clinical improvement |
| **Mastoiditis, chronic** | Antibiotics only for acute superinfections (according to culture of drainage); also, when chronic *Pseudomonas* infection, ticarcillin 200–300 mg/kg/day IV div q4–6h × 5–7 days OR other antipseudomonal beta-lactam | Daily cleansing of ear important; After resolution, use amoxicillin or sulfa prophylaxis for otitis; If no response, surgery |
| **Sinusitis, acute** (*H. influenzae*, non–type b, pneumococcus, streptococcus, *Moraxella*) | Same as for acute otitis media but 14–21 days may be needed | Sinus irrigations when indicated |

E. NOSE AND OROPHARYNGEAL INFECTIONS

| | | |
|---|---|---|
| **Dental abscess** | Clindamycin 30 mg/kg/day PO, IV, IM div q6–8h OR penicillin G 100,000 U/kg/day IV div q6h | Usually oral aerobes and anaerobes; tooth extraction may be necessary |
| **Diphtheria** | Erythromycin 40–50 mg/kg/day PO div q6h × 14 days OR penicillin G 150,000 U/kg/day IV div q6h; PLUS antitoxin | Antitoxin available only from CDC [(404) 639-2889]; Isolation until 3 daily nose and throat cultures negative |

| Clinical Diagnosis | Therapy | Comments |
|---|---|---|
| **Streptococcal tonsillopharyngitis, scarlet fever and peritonsillar cellulitis** | Penicillin V 25–50 mg/kg/day PO div q6–8h × 10 days OR benzathine penicillin 25,000 U/kg IM (max 1.2 million U) as a single dose; Erythromycin or clindamycin for penicillin-allergic patients | Alternatives: In practice, amoxicillin and cephalosporins are more commonly used than penicillin |
| **Epiglottitis** (aryepiglottitis, supraglottitis) | Cefuroxime 100–150 mg/kg/day IV, IM div q8h OR chloramphenicol 50–75 mg/kg/day IV div q6h × 5–7 days | Provide airway; *H. influenzae* type b in unimmunized infants |
| **Bacterial tracheitis** (staphylococcal, streptococcal, pneumococcal, *Haemophilus*) | Oxacillin 150 mg/kg/day IV div q6h or cefazolin 100 mg/kg/day IV div q8h AND cefotaxime 150 mg/kg/day div q8h or ceftriaxone 50 mg/kg/day q24h; Alternative: cefuroxime 100–150 mg/kg/day div q8h | May represent bacterial superinfection of viral laryngotracheobronchitis |
| **Gingivostomatitis, herpetic** | Acyclovir 15 mg/kg PO five times daily × 7 days (Give IV for severe disease) | Regimen reported effective in one study |
| **Retropharyngeal or lateral pharyngeal cellulitis or abscess** (Mixed aerobic and anaerobic infection) | Clindamycin 30 mg/kg/day PO, IV, IM div q6h OR oxacillin 150 mg/kg/day IV div q6h or cefazolin 100 mg/kg/day IV div q8h AND cefotaxime 150 mg/kg/day IV div q8h or ceftriaxone 50 mg/kg/day IV q24h | I&D when pus present; Consider tonsillectomy for peritonsillar abscess; Possible airway compromise/mediastinitis |

## F. LOWER RESPIRATORY INFECTIONS

| Clinical Diagnosis | Therapy | Comments |
|---|---|---|
| **Abscess, lung** | | |
| - Primary, putrid (i.e., foul-smelling) | Clindamycin 30 mg/kg/day PO, IM, IV div q6–8h × 10 days or longer; Ticarcillin/clavulanate or meropenem may be useful alternatives | Usually polymicrobial infection with aerobes and anaerobes |

| | | |
|---|---|---|
| - Primary, nonputrid | Cefuroxime 100–150 mg/kg/day IV, IM div q8h or other beta-lactamase–resistant beta-lactam; × 10 days or longer | Bronchoscopy necessary if abscess fails to drain; Surgical excision rarely necessary |
| - Secondary to other focus of infection (osteomyelitis, etc.) | Oxacillin 150 mg/kg/day IV div q6h <u>OR</u> cefazolin 100 mg/kg/day IV div q8h; × 10 days or longer <u>OR</u> other beta-lactams | Usually staphylococcal; Cephalosporin for coliforms |
| **Allergic bronchopulmonary aspergillosis** | Prednisone 0.5 mg/kg every other day | Larger dosages may lead to tissue invasion |
| **Bronchitis, acute** | No antibiotic for most cases (viral); if bacterial infection suspected, use same drugs as for acute otitis or sinusitis (See page 24) | *Haemophilus*, *Moraxella*, pneumococcus most common pathogens in adults and (?) in children |
| **Cystic fibrosis, acute exacerbation** | Ticarcillin 300–400 mg/kg/day IV div q4h <u>AND</u> tobramycin 6–10 mg/kg/day IM, IV div q6–8h; Alternatives: other anti-*Pseudomonas* beta-lactams and aminoglycosides <u>OR</u> ciprofloxacin 30 mg/kg/day PO, IV div q8h; × 7–10 days | Larger than normal dosages of aminoglycosides required in most patients with CF; Monitor peak serum concentrations of aminoglycosides |
| **Pertussis** | Erythromycin (estolate may be preferable) 50 mg/kg/day PO div q6h; × 14 days (Re-administer vomited doses, or change to ampicillin 100 mg/kg/day IV, IM div q6h) | Hospitalize young babies; Avoid mist therapy; Avoid cough suppressants; Isolate for the first 5 days of therapy |
| **Pneumonia: Bronchopneumonia** | | |
| - Mild to moderate illness | No antibiotic therapy unless epidemiological or clinical reasons to suspect specific pathogen other than virus | Most viral; Broad spectrum antibiotics increase risk of superinfection |

| Clinical Diagnosis | Therapy | Comments |
|---|---|---|
| **Bronchopneumonia** (cont.) | | |
| - Serious, life-threatening illness (Pneumococcus, group A streptococcus, *S. aureus* or atypical pneumonia pathogens) | Initially, until etiology established, oxacillin 150 mg/kg/day IV div q6h AND gentamicin 6–7.5 mg/kg/day IM, IV div q8h, OR cefotaxime or cefuroxime 150 mg/kg/day IV div q8h | Tracheal aspirate or bronchoalveolar lavage for Gram's stain and culture when indicated; Consider a macrolide for atypical pneumonia |
| **Pneumonia: Lobar or segmental consolidation** | | Consider *H. influenzae* type b in the unimmunized child |
| - Pneumococcal, initial therapy or penicillin-nonsusceptible, or unknown etiology | Cefuroxime 100–150 mg/kg/day IV, IM div q8h; OR ceftriaxone 50 mg/kg/day IV, IM q24h; × 10 days (Alternative: clindamycin for susceptible strains) | Consider adding vancomycin for highly penicillin-resistant strains; Change to PO after improvement (decreased fever, no oxygen needed) |
| - Pneumococcal, penicillin-susceptible | Penicillin G 150,000 U/kg/day IV div q4–6h × 10 days | Change to PO penicillin V 50–75 mg/kg/day, div q6–8h after improvement |
| - *Klebsiella pneumoniae* | Cefotaxime 150 mg/kg/day IV, IM div q8h; OR ceftriaxone 50 mg/kg/day IV, IM q24h (Alternative: gentamicin 6–7.5 mg/kg/day IM, IV div q8h × 10 days or longer OR amikacin 15–20 mg/kg/ day IM, IV div q8h) | Suspect if distended lobe; Abscesses common but empyema rare |
| **Pneumonia: With empyema** | | Initial therapy based on Gram's stain of empyema fluid; Consider *H. influenzae* type b in the unimmunized child |
| - Group A streptococcal | Penicillin G 150,000 U/kg/day IV div q4–6h × 10 days (Change to PO penicillin V 50–75 mg/kg/day, div q6–8h after clinical improvement); | Closed chest tube drainage of purulent fluid; Typically clinical improvement is slow |

| | | |
|---|---|---|
| - Pneumococcal | (See above) | Definitive therapy is based on susceptibility of strain |
| - Staphylococcal | Oxacillin 150 mg/kg/day IV div q6h <u>OR</u> vancomycin 40 mg/kg/day div q6h; × 21 days or longer (Alternatives: 1st generation cephalosporins) | Closed chest tube drainage of empyema; consider adding gentamicin for synergy |
| **- Pneumonia: Immunosuppressed, neutropenic host**<br>- *Staphylococcus aureus*<br>- *Pseudomonas aeruginosa*<br>- Enteric Gram-negative bacilli | Oxacillin 150 mg/kg/day IV div q6h <u>OR</u> cefazolin 100 mg/kg/day IV div q8h <u>OR</u> vancomycin 40 mg/kg/day IV div q6h (if methicillin-resistant *Staphylococcus* suspected) <u>AND</u> ceftazidime 150 mg/kg/day IV div q8h; Alternative: oxacillin (as above) <u>AND</u> mezlocillin or ticarcillin 200–300 mg/kg/day IV div q6h <u>AND</u> amikacin 15–22.5 mg/kg/day or gentamicin 6–7.5 mg/kg/day IM, IV div q8h | Consider opportunistic bacteria, *Pneumocystis*, cytomegalovirus, fungi, tuberculosis; Biopsy or bronchoalveolar lavage of lung may be needed to establish diagnosis |
| **- Pneumonia: Interstitial pneumonia syndrome of early infancy** | Supportive, or (if chlamydia suspected) erythromycin 40 mg/kg/day PO div q6h; × 14 days | Most viral or chlamydial; Role of *Ureaplasma* uncertain |
| **Other pneumonias of established etiology** | | |
| - *Chlamydia pneumoniae* (TWAR), *C. psittaci* or *C. trachomatis* | A macrolide <u>OR</u> tetracycline (patients > 7 yrs) (ampicillin for *C. trachomatis*) | For dosage, see Section VIII |
| - Cytomegalovirus | Ganciclovir (plus IVIG) | For dosage, see Section VIII |

| Clinical Diagnosis | Therapy | Comments |
|---|---|---|
| **Pneumonia** (cont.) | | |
| - *Escherichia coli*, *Enterobacter* spp. | An aminoglycoside or cephalosporin (2nd or 3rd generation for *E. coli*, 3rd or 4th generation for *Enterobacter* spp.) | For dosage, see Section VIII |
| - *Francisella tularensis* | Gentamicin or streptomycin | (See page 48) |
| - Fungi | Amphotericin B or combined therapy | For dosage, see Section VI |
| - Influenza A | Amantadine or rimantadine | For dosage, see page 41 |
| - Legionnaires' disease | A macrolide and rifampin | For dosage, see Section VIII |
| - Melioidosis | (See page 42) | |
| - *Mycoplasma pneumoniae* | A macrolide or tetracycline | For dosage, see Section VIII |
| - *Paragonimus westermani* | Praziquantel | For dosage, see page 63 |
| - *Pneumocystis carinii* pneumonia | (See page 58) | |
| - *P. aeruginosa* | Anti-*Pseudomonas* beta-lactam antibiotic, ± an aminoglycoside | For dosage, see Section VIII |
| - Respiratory syncytial virus infection (bronchiolitis, pneumonia) | Ribavirin 6-g vial (20 mg/ml in sterile water) aerosolized by SPAG-2 generator over 18- to 20-hr period daily × 3–5 days | Treat only for severe disease or patients with underlying cardiopulmonary disease |

| | | |
|---|---|---|
| **Tuberculosis** | | |
| - Primary pulmonary disease | Isoniazid 10–15 mg/kg/day (max 300 mg) PO, IM × 6–9 mos AND rifampin 10–20 mg/kg/day (max 600 mg) PO, IV × 6–9 mos AND pyrazinamide 20–40 mg/kg/day PO × 2 mos; If in area with known drug resistance, add ethambutol 20 mg/kg/day PO OR streptomycin 30 mg/kg/day IM initially | Test for HIV infection; Directly observed therapy (DOT) preferred; After 1 month of therapy, can change to twice weekly dosing (Double dosage of INH and PYR; rifampin remains same dosage) |
| - Skin test conversion (subclinical infection) | Isoniazid 10–15 mg/kg/day (max 300 mg) PO daily × 6–9 mos (12 mos for immune compromised patients) | Single drug Rx if no clinical or radiographic evidence of disease |
| - Exposed infant < 4 yrs, or immunocompromised patient | Isoniazid 10–15 mg/kg PO daily × 3 mos after last exposure | If PPD remains negative and child well, stop prophylaxis |
| G. HEART INFECTIONS | | |
| **Endocarditis** | | |
| - Viridans streptococcus | Penicillin G 150,000 U/kg/day IV div q4–6h × 30 days; OR penicillin AND gentamicin 6–7.5 mg/kg/day IM, IV div q8h × 14 days; OR vancomycin 40 mg/kg/day IV div q6h OR ceftriaxone 50 mg/kg/day IV, IM q24h × 30 days | For nutritionally deficient streptococci, use vancomycin |
| - Enterococcus | Ampicillin 150 mg/kg/day IV, IM div q6h × 30 days AND gentamicin 6–7.5 mg/kg/day IM, IV div q8h; OR penicillin G 250,000 U/kg/day IV div q4–6h AND streptomycin 30 mg/kg/day IM div q12h; × 30 days | Longest experience with the penicillin-streptomycin regimen; Combined Rx used for synergistic bactericidal activity |

| Clinical Diagnosis | Therapy | Comments |
|---|---|---|
| **Endocarditis** (cont.) | | |
| - *Staphylococcus aureus, Staphylococcus epidermidis* | Nafcillin or oxacillin 150 mg/kg/day IV div q6h × 6 wks OR, for methicillin-resistant staphylococci, vancomycin 40 mg/kg/day IV div q6h; Consider adding rifampin or aminoglycoside for synergistic effect | Surgery may be necessary in acute phase; Avoid cephalosporins because of conflicting data on efficacy |
| - Pneumococcus, gonococcus, Group A streptococcus | Penicillin G 150,000 U/kg/day IV div q4–6h × 30 days (vancomycin, cefotaxime or ceftriaxone for penicillin-resistant pneumococci) | Ceftriaxone for gonococcus until susceptibilities known |
| - Prophylaxis for: | | |
| - Dental, esophageal and upper respiratory procedures | Amoxicillin PO 50 mg/kg 1 hr before procedure OR Ampicillin IM, IV 50 mg/kg 30 min before procedure | **If penicillin allergy:** Azithromycin or clarithromycin PO 15 mg/kg 1 hr before clindamycin 20 mg/kg 30 min before (IV) or 60 min before (PO) |
| - Genitourinary and gastro-intestinal procedures | Ampicillin IM, IV 50 mg/kg AND gentamicin IM, IV 1.5 mg/kg 30 min before; 6 hr later ampicillin IM, IV 25 mg/kg | Vancomycin IV 20 mg/kg over 1–2 hr AND gentamicin IM, IV |
| **Purulent pericarditis** | | SURGICAL DRAINAGE OF PUS |
| - *S. aureus* | Oxacillin 150 mg/kg/day IV div q6h OR cefazolin 100 mg/kg/day IV div q8h OR (for methicillin-resistant staphylococci) vancomycin 40 mg/kg/day IV div q6h; × 3 wks or longer | Change to penicillin G if susceptible |

| | | |
|---|---|---|
| - *H. influenzae* b | Cefuroxime 100–150 mg/kg/day IV, IM div q8h × 10–14 days; Alternatives: cefotaxime, ceftriaxone | Ampicillin for beta-lactamase–negative strains |
| - Pneumococcus, meningococcus, group A streptococcus | Penicillin G 150,000 U/kg/day IV, IM div q4–6h × 10–14 days | Ceftriaxone, cefotaxime, or vancomycin for penicillin-resistant pneumococci |
| - Coliform bacilli | Cefotaxime 100–150 mg/kg/day IV, IM div q6–8h × 3 wks or longer; Alternatives: other cephalosporins, aminoglycoside | Alternative drugs depending on susceptibilities |
| - Tuberculous | (See page 31) | Corticosteroids for first 2–3 mos |
| H. <u>GASTROINTESTINAL INFECTIONS</u> (***See Section VII for parasitic infections***) | | |
| ***Helicobacter pylori* gastritis, peptic ulcer disease** | Clarithromycin 500 mg PO t.i.d. <u>AND</u> amoxicillin 1 g PO twice daily <u>AND</u> omeprazole 40 mg PO once daily × 2 wks, followed by omeprazole alone × 2 wks (adult dosage) | Most data from studies in adults; Other regimens include bismuth, amoxicillin, metronidazole |
| **Shigellosis** | Cefixime 8 mg/kg/day PO div 12–24 hrs × 5 days <u>OR</u> TMP/SMX 8 mg/kg/day of TMP component PO div q12h <u>OR</u> (for patients > 18 yrs) ciprofloxacin 500 mg PO q12h | Ampicillin when *Shigella* susceptible; Avoid antiperistaltic drugs; Treat to decrease communicability, even if symptoms resolving |

| Clinical Diagnosis | Therapy | Comments |
| --- | --- | --- |
| **Salmonellosis** | Usually none for self-limited diarrhea OR amoxicillin 50 mg/kg/day PO div q8h × 5–7 days OR TMP/SMX as for shigellosis (See page 43 for typhoid fever) | Treat infants with bacteremia, compromised hosts, and those with septic clinical picture or colitis (IV antibiotics for bacteremia) |
| ***Escherichia coli*** | | |

**A Note on *E. coli* and Diarrheal Disease:** Antibiotic susceptibility of *E. coli* varies considerably from region to region in the world. For mild to moderate disease, TMP/SMX may be started as initial therapy; for severe disease, cefixime may be used; cultures and antibiotic susceptibility testing are recommended for significant disease.

| Clinical Diagnosis | Therapy | Comments |
| --- | --- | --- |
| - Enteropathogenic | Neomycin 100 mg/kg/day PO div q6–8h | Most traditional "enteropathogenic" strains not toxigenic or invasive |
| - Enterotoxigenic (traveler's diarrhea) | Trimethoprim-sulfamethoxazole or cefixime (as for shigellosis) | Most illnesses brief and self-limited |
| - Enteroinvasive | (?) Orally absorbable antibiotic, such as ampicillin, amoxicillin or TMP/SMX | No controlled clinical trials on which to base a recommendation |
| ***Yersinia enterocolitica*** | Antimicrobial therapy probably not of value | May mimic appendicitis (most strains are susceptible to TMP/SMX or 3rd generation cephalosporin, but limited clinical data exist) |
| ***Campylobacter jejuni*** | Erythromycin 40 mg/kg/day PO div q6h × 5 days; Alternative (for adults): ciprofloxacin | Abdominal pain may mimic acute surgical abdomen |
| ***Aeromonas* sp.** | (?) TMP/SMX as for shigellosis | Efficacy not established |

| | | |
|---|---|---|
| **Antibiotic-associated colitis** | Metronidazole 30 mg/kg/day PO div q6h; Alternative: vancomycin 40 mg/kg/day PO div q6h × 7 days | Due to overgrowth of *C. difficile* in gut; Vancomycin may cause emergence of resistant enterococci in gut |
| **Perirectal abscess** | Clindamycin 30–40 mg/kg/day IV, PO div q6–8h AND aminoglycoside or cephalosporin | *S. aureus* common but may be mixed with coliforms, anaerobes; Surgical drainage |

I. GENITOURINARY AND SEXUALLY TRANSMITTED INFECTIONS

Consider testing for HIV infection in children with sexually transmitted diseases; consider sexual abuse in prepubertal children with STDs.

| | | |
|---|---|---|
| **Genital herpes infection** | Acyclovir 400 mg PO 3 × daily × 5 days (recurrent episode) OR acyclovir 200 mg PO 5 × daily × 7–10 days (first episode) OR (for severe disease) acyclovir 15 mg/kg/day as 1 hr IV infusion div q8h × 5–7 days | Most effective when started early in course of infection; For prevention of recurrence 400 mg twice daily |
| **Urinary tract infection** | | |
| - Acute cystitis (*E. coli*) | TMP/SMX 8 mg/kg/day of TMP component PO div q12h for mild to moderate disease, OR cefixime 8 mg/kg/day PO div 12–24 hrs OR (for patients > 18 yrs) ciprofloxacin 500 mg PO q12h for initial therapy of more severe disease (Alternative: amoxicillin 30 mg/kg/day PO div q8h if susceptible); × 7–10 days | *In vivo* susceptibility test: follow-up culture after 36–48 hrs treatment; If culture positive, change treatment according to *in vitro* susceptibilities |
| - Acute pyelonephritis (*E. coli*) | Ceftriaxone 50 mg/kg/day IV, IM q24h OR gentamicin 6 mg/kg/day IV, IM div q8h OR TMP/SMX 8 mg/kg/day of TMP component PO, IV div q12h; × 10 days | Parenteral drug if sepsis suspected; Change to appropriate oral drug after clinical response |
| - Prophylaxis for recurrent bacteriuria | TMP/SMX 2 mg TMP–10 mg SMX/kg PO q1–2 days OR nitrofurantoin 1–2 mg/kg PO q1–2 days at bedtime | Prophylaxis for patients with reflux or frequent infections; Resistance eventually develops to any antibiotic used |

| Clinical Diagnosis | Therapy | Comments |
|---|---|---|
| **Epididymitis** | Cefuroxime 100–150 mg/kg/day div q8h OR nafcillin 150 mg/kg/day IV div q6h and chloramphenicol 50–75 mg/kg/day IV, PO div q6h; × 7–10 days | Usually due to *Haemophilus* or *S. aureus* in young children; Treat as for gonorrhea and chlamydia in older children |
| **Trichomoniasis** | See Section VII | |
| **Vaginitis or cervicitis** | | |
| - Vulvovaginal candidiasis | See Section VI | |
| - *Shigella* | As for diarrhea (See page 33) | 50% have bloody discharge; Usually not associated with diarrhea |
| - Group A streptococcus | Penicillin V 50–75 mg/kg/day PO div q6–8h × 10 days | |
| - Chlamydial | Doxycycline (patients > 7 yrs) 4 mg/kg/day (max 200 mg) PO div q12h × 7 days OR azithromycin 1 g PO as single dose | Alternatives: erythromycin, sulfisoxazole, amoxicillin |
| - Bacterial vaginosis (formerly "nonspecific vaginitis") | Metronidazole 500 mg PO twice daily × 7 days or as single 2 g PO dose; Alternative: intravaginal clindamycin cream or metronidazole gel | Caused by synergy of *Gardnerella* with anaerobes |
| **Gonorrhea** | | |
| - Newborns | See Section III | |

| | | |
|---|---|---|
| - Genital infections | Ceftriaxone 125 mg IM OR cefixime 400 mg PO OR azithromycin 2 g PO (each as a single dose); Treatment regimens of demonstrated efficacy for children:<br>1) Procaine penicillin G 100,000 U/kg IM (max 4.8 mU) as single dose (two injection sites) AND probenecid 25 mg/kg PO (max 1 g)<br>2) Amoxicillin 50 mg/kg PO as single dose AND probenecid 25 mg/kg PO<br>3) Spectinomycin 40 mg/kg IM as single dose | Ceftriaxone preferred; Serologic test for syphilis; Repeat in 3 mos if treated with something other than penicillin; Follow with treatment for presumed chlamydia |
| - Disseminated gonococcal infection | Ceftriaxone 50 mg/kg/day IM, IV once daily × 7 days | No studies in children: Increase dosage for meningitis |
| **Syphilis** | | See most recent CDC *Sexually Transmitted Diseases Treatment Guidelines* |
| - Congenital | See Section III | |
| - Primary, secondary | Benzathine penicillin G 2,400,000 U IM (approximately 50,000 U/kg) in two injection sites, single dose OR doxycycline 4 mg/kg/day (max 200 mg) PO div q12h × 14 days (patients > 7 yrs) | Follow-up serologic tests at 3, 6, and 12 mos; Do not use benzathine-procaine penicillin mixtures |
| - Syphilis of more than 1 yr duration | Benzathine penicillin G 2,400,000 U IM (approximately 50,000 U/kg) in two injection sites weekly for three doses | Optimal treatment schedule not established; For CNS syphilis, consider use of either crystalline penicillin G or procaine penicillin to achieve adequate CSF concentrations |

| Clinical Diagnosis | Therapy | Comments |
|---|---|---|
| **Syphilis** (cont.) | | |
| **Chancroid** | Ceftriaxone 250 mg IM as single dose OR erythromycin 2 g/day PO div q6h × 7 days OR azithromycin 1 g PO as single dose | Serologic test for syphilis |
| **Lymphogranuloma venereum** (*Chlamydia trachomatis*) | Doxycycline 4 mg/kg/day (max 200 mg) PO (patients > 7 yrs) div q12h OR erythromycin 2 g/day PO div q6h; × 21 days | |
| **Pelvic inflammatory disease** | Cefoxitin 2 g IV q6h and doxycycline 100 mg PO bid OR clindamycin 900 mg IV q8h and gentamicin 1.5 mg/kg IV, IM q8h (Other regimens include oxacillin, ciprofloxacin, metronidazole) | Two drugs given until clinical improvement and followed by doxycycline alone to complete 14 days |

## J. CENTRAL NERVOUS SYSTEM INFECTIONS

NOTE: **In areas where penicillin-resistant pneumococci exist, initial empiric therapy should be with vancomycin plus cefotaxime or ceftriaxone until susceptibility test results are available.**

**Bacterial meningitis**

NOTE: Dexamethasone (0.6 mg/kg/day IV div q6h × 4 days) as an adjunct to antibiotic therapy decreases hearing deficits and possibly other neurologic sequelae in *Haemophilus* meningitis and possibly other types. The first dose of dexamethasone is preferably given before the first dose of antibiotic.

| Clinical Diagnosis | Therapy | Comments |
|---|---|---|
| - Neonatal | See Section III | |
| - *H. influenzae* type b | Cefotaxime 200–300 mg/kg/day IV div q6h OR ceftriaxone either 100 mg/kg/day IV div q12h or q24h; Alternative: ampicillin 200–400 mg/kg/day IV div q6h OR chloramphenicol 100 mg/kg/day IV div q6h; × 10 days | Chloramphenicol can be given PO; Rifampin prophylaxis for patients and unimmunized contacts (for susceptible strains) according to Red Book recommendations |

| | | |
|---|---|---|
| - *Pneumococcus* | For penicillin-resistant pneumococci use vancomycin 60 mg/kg/day IV div q6h plus cefotaxime or ceftriaxone (as above) OR (for susceptible strains) Penicillin G 250,000 U/kg/day IV div q4h; × 10 days | Some pneumococci resistant to penicillin but susceptible to cefotaxime and ceftriaxone may be treated with these antibiotics |
| - *Meningococcus* (including meningococcemia) | Penicillin G 250,000 U/kg/day IV div q4h × 7 days; Regimens given for *Haemophilus* are effective for meningococcal infection; Rare strains are resistant to penicillin | Meningococcal prophylaxis: rifampin 10 mg/kg PO q12h × four doses OR ceftriaxone 125–250 mg IM once OR ciprofloxacin 500 mg PO once (adults) |
| - Unknown bacterial | Vancomycin AND cefotaxime or ceftriaxone (as above) | Other approved drugs: ceftazidime, ceftizoxime, meropenem |
| - Tuberculous | Isoniazid 15 mg/kg/day PO, IM div q12–24h AND rifampin 15 mg/kg/day, IV, PO div q12–24h × 12 mos AND streptomycin 30 mg/kg/day IM div q12h for first 4 wks of therapy AND pyrazinamide 30 mg/kg/day PO div q12–24h for first 2 mos | Hyponatremia from inappropriate ADH common; Ventricular drainage may be necessary; Steroids suppress symptoms and may improve prognosis |
| **Shunt infections** | | |
| - *S. epidermidis* or *S. aureus* | Vancomycin 60 mg/kg/day IV div q6h OR nafcillin 150–200 mg/kg/day (?) PLUS an aminoglycoside or rifampin; × 10–14 days | Surgery for shunt removal usually necessary; May be synergy between antibiotics |
| - Coliform bacilli | Cefotaxime 200–300 mg/kg/day IV div q6h OR ampicillin 200–400 mg/kg/day IV div q6h AND gentamicin 6–7.5 mg/kg/day or amikacin 15–20 mg/kg/day IV, IM div q8h; × 21 days or longer | Select appropriate drug based on *in vitro* susceptibilities; Meropenem may be effective for cefotaxime-resistant strains |

| Clinical Diagnosis | Therapy | Comments |
|---|---|---|
| **Brain abscess** | Until etiology established nafcillin or vancomycin (as for meningitis) AND cefotaxime (as for meningitis) AND metronidazole 30 mg/kg/day IV, PO div q8h; × 7–10 days after surgery; Longer therapy if no surgery | Surgery; Anaerobes common; Add anti-*Pseudomonas* drug if secondary to chronic otitis; Follow abscess size with CT scans |
| **Herpes simplex encephalitis** | Acyclovir 30 mg/kg/day as 1 hr or longer IV infusion div q8h × 21 days | (See Newborn section) |
| **Toxoplasma encephalitis** | See Section VII | |

K. MISCELLANEOUS SYSTEMIC INFECTIONS

| Clinical Diagnosis | Therapy | Comments |
|---|---|---|
| **Actinomycosis** | Penicillin G 250,000 U/kg/day IV div q4h until improved; Thereafter penicillin V 100 mg/kg/day PO div q6h × several mos | Surgery as indicated; Tetracycline for penicillin-allergic |
| **Brucellosis** | Tetracycline 40 mg/kg/day PO, div q6h OR doxycycline 4 mg/kg IV once daily (patients > 7 yrs); TMP 10 mg/kg-SMX 50 mg/kg/day PO div q12h if < 7 yrs; Rifampin (15–20 mg/kg/day div q12h) given as second drug; × 4–6 wks | Add gentamicin 6–7.5 mg/kg/day IV, IM div q8h for the first wk for serious disease |
| **Cat-scratch disease** | Supportive; Aspiration of pus; In one study, azithromycin was beneficial | Aminoglycosides, rifampin, TMP/SMX, ciprofloxacin, cefotaxime may be effective |
| **Chickenpox/Shingles** | Acyclovir 80 mg/kg/day PO div q6h × 5–7 days, when indicated (Most cases do not require therapy) | Parenteral therapy for severe cases (See Varicella-zoster, disseminated, page 43) |
| **Ehrlichiosis** (human monocytic or granulocytic) | (See Rickettsial infection, page 43) | |

| | | |
|---|---|---|
| **Febrile neutropenic patient** | Oxacillin or cefazolin (or vancomycin if methicillin resistant *Staphylococcus* is suspected) AND anti-*Pseudomonas* beta-lactam AND aminoglycoside; OR cefepime | If no response in 5–7 days and no bacterial etiology demonstrated, consider empiric antifungal therapy with amphotericin B; Dosages in Section VIII |
| **Human immunodeficiency virus infection** | Initial therapy with three (or more) drugs including a protease inhibitor; Consult with HIV expert because new information about optimal regimens is constantly emerging | (See page 8 for prophylaxis for newborns) |
| **Infant botulism** | Botulism immune globulin (BIG) 50 mg/kg IV × 1 [Obtained from the California State Health Department: (510) 540-2646]; Trivalent antitoxin for food-borne or wound botulism; Aminoglycosides potentiate effect of toxin | BIG is very expensive; ICU supportive therapy; Giving enemas to remove constipated stool and toxin is controversial; Antibiotics may facilitate cell death and release of toxin |
| **Influenza A infection** | Amantadine 5 mg/kg/day (max 200 mg) PO div q12h OR rimantadine 5 mg/kg/day (max 200 mg) PO div once or twice daily × 7 days; Ribavirin aerosol (as for RSV infection, page 30) may be effective | Treat within 48–72 hrs of onset; Rx especially for high-risk patients |
| **Kawasaki syndrome** | No antibiotics; IV gamma globulin 2 g/kg as single dose; may need to repeat dose for persisting fever | Aspirin 80 mg/kg/day div q6h in acute, febrile phase; Then, initiate low dosage (3–5 mg/kg/day) aspirin Rx for 6–8 wks, or until the platelet count and ESR are normal |
| **Leprosy** | Dapsone 100 mg PO and clofazimine 50 mg PO daily OR rifampin 600 mg PO and clofazimine 300 mg PO monthly; × 2–6 yrs (adult dosages) | Consult CDC for advice about treatment |
| **Leptospirosis** | Penicillin G 250,000 U/kg/day IV, IM div q4–6h OR tetracycline 40 mg/kg/day PO div q6h; × 7–10 days | |

| Clinical Diagnosis | Therapy | Comments |
|---|---|---|
| **Lyme disease** | Early disease: Doxycycline 4 mg/kg/day PO div q12h (patients > 7 yrs) OR amoxicillin 40 mg/kg/day (max 3 g) (?) with probenecid 25 mg/kg/day (max 1500) PO div q8h; × 14–21 days | Late disease: ceftriaxone 100 (CNS) or 50 (others) mg/kg once daily IM, IV × 14–21 days |
| **Measles** | Supportive therapy; Ribavirin has been used 15 mg/kg/day IV div q8h × 10 days (double dose on first day); Vitamin A therapy reported to be beneficial in malnourished patients | Consider ribavirin in severe disease/ compromised host (IV formulation not commercially available) |
| **Melioidosis** | Acute sepsis: Ceftazidime 120 mg/kg/day IV div q8h OR chloramphenicol 50–75 mg/kg/day IV, PO div q6h AND sulfisoxazole 120–150 mg/kg/day PO div q6h AND an aminoglycoside; × 10–14 days | Ceftazidime more effective than conventional three-drug therapy in one study |
| | Chronic infection: Trimethoprim-sulfamethoxazole 8 mg TMP/kg–40 mg SMX/kg/day div q12h × several wks | Tetracycline for children > 7 yrs of age |
| **Mycobacteriosis** (Disseminated MAI disease in compromised host) | Usually treated with four or five drugs (e.g., ciprofloxacin, clofazimine, ethambutol, rifampin, amikacin, clarithromycin) | See Section VIII for dosage |
| **Nocardiosis** | Sulfisoxazole 120–150 mg/kg/day PO div q6h × 6 wks or longer; For severe infection, amikacin 15–20 mg/kg/day IM, IV div q8h | Surgery when indicated; Trimethoprim-sulfamethoxazole or cycloserine as alternatives |
| **Peritonitis** | | |
| - Primary | Penicillin G 150,000 U/kg/day IV div q4h; × 7–10 days | Usually pneumococcal; Other antibiotics according to culture and susceptibility tests |

| | | |
|---|---|---|
| - Secondary to bowel perforation or appendicitis (Enteric Gram-negative bacilli, *Bacteroides* sp., *Enterococcus* sp.) | Meropenem 60 mg/kg/day IV div q8h <u>OR</u> clindamycin 30 mg/kg/day IV, IM div q6h plus gentamicin 6–7.5 mg/kg/day IV, IM div q8h × 10 days or longer | Many other regimens claimed to be effective |
| - Secondary to peritoneal dialysis | Antibiotic added to dialysate in concentrations approximating those attained in serum for systemic disease (e.g., 8 μg/ml for gentamicin; 50 μg/ml for vancomycin, etc.) | Selection of antibiotic based on organism isolated from peritoneal fluid; Systemic antibiotics if there is accompanying bacteremia |
| **Rickettsial infection** | Tetracycline 40 mg/kg/day PO div q6h <u>OR</u> chloramphenicol 50–75 mg/kg/day IV div q6h; × 10–14 days | Tetracycline is preferred for all ages, as it appears to be the most effective therapy and one treatment course is unlikely to cause significant tooth or bone alterations |
| **Tetanus** | Metronidazole 30 mg/kg/day IV, PO div q6h <u>OR</u> penicillin G 100,000 U/kg/day IV div q4–6h; × 10 days | Plus antitoxin and sedation |
| **Toxic shock syndrome** | Nafcillin or oxacillin 150 mg/kg/day IV div q6h <u>OR</u> cefazolin 100 mg/kg/day IV div q8h; × 7 days | General supportive care of prime importance; (?) Add clindamycin to decrease toxin production and IVIG to bind circulating toxin |
| **Tularemia** | Gentamicin 6–7.5 mg/kg/day IM, IV div q8h <u>OR</u> streptomycin 30 mg/kg/day IM div q12h; × 7–10 days (Dosage of streptomycin may be reduced by one-half after 3 days) | Tetracycline less effective alternative |
| **Typhoid fever** | Ceftriaxone 50 mg/kg/day q24h <u>OR</u> cefotaxime 150 mg/kg/day div q8h <u>OR</u> amoxicillin (for susceptible strains) 100 mg/kg/day PO div q8h; × 14 days | TMP/SMX may also be effective |
| **Varicella-zoster, disseminated** (compromised host) | Acyclovir 1500 mg/m$^2$/day (approximately 45 mg/kg/day) IV as 1- to 2-hr infusion div q8h; × 5–7 days | Also used for severe or complicated chickenpox in normal host; Alternatives: famciclovir, foscarnet |

## V. PREFERRED THERAPY FOR SPECIFIC BACTERIAL AND VIRAL PATHOGENS

NOTES: 1. For fungal and parasitic infections see Sections VI and VII, respectively.
2. Limitations of space do not permit listing of all possible alternative antimicrobials.

| Organism | Clinical Illness | Drug of Choice | Alternatives |
|---|---|---|---|
| *Acinetobacter baumanii* | Sepsis, meningitis | Meropenem | An aminoglycoside; A fluoroquinolone; anti-*Pseudomonas* beta-lactam; TMP/SMX |
| *Actinobacillus actinomycetem-comitans* | Abscesses, endocarditis | Ampicillin | Tetracycline (patients > 7 yrs); Chloramphenicol |
| *Actinomyces israelii* | Actinomycosis | Penicillin G | Tetracycline (patients > 7 yrs); Ampicillin; Clindamycin |
| *Aeromonas* spp. | Diarrhea, sepsis, cellulitis | TMP/SMX | An aminoglycoside; Meropenem |
| *Arcanobacterium haemolyticum* | Pharyngitis | A macrolide | Penicillin G; A 1st generation cephalosporin |
| *Bacillus anthracis* | Anthrax | Penicillin G | A macrolide; Tetracycline (patients > 7 yrs) |
| *Bacillus cereus* or *subtilis* | Sepsis | Vancomycin | Clindamycin; Meropenem |
| *Bacteroides fragilis* | Peritonitis, sepsis, abscesses | Clindamycin; Metroni-dazole for CNS infection | Cefoxitin; Anti-*Pseudomonas* penicillins; Meropenem |
| *Bacteroides,* other spp. | Pneumonia, sepsis, abscesses | Penicillin G or ampicillin | Clindamycin; Chloramphenicol; Metro-nidazole |

| | | | |
|---|---|---|---|
| *Bartonella bacilliformis* | Bartonellosis | Chloramphenicol; Tetracycline (patients > 7 yrs) | Penicillin G |
| *Bartonella henselae* | Cat-scratch disease | Azithromycin; TMP/SMX; Gentamicin | Rifampin; A fluoroquinolone |
| | Bacillary angiomatosis, peliosis hepatis | A macrolide | Tetracycline (patients > 7 yrs) |
| *Bordetella holmesii* | Sepsis | Ceftriaxone | Unknown |
| *Bordetella pertussis, parapertussis* | Pertussis | A macrolide | TMP/SMX; Ampicillin |
| *Borrelia* spp. | Relapsing fever, Lyme disease | Tetracycline (patients > 7 yrs) | Penicillin G; A 3rd generation cephalosporin; A macrolide |
| *Brucella* spp. | Brucellosis | Tetracycline (patients > 7 yrs) + gentamicin | TMP/SMX; Rifampin |
| *Burkholderia cepacia* | Pneumonia, sepsis | TMP/SMX + ceftazidime | Doxycycline; Chloramphenicol |
| *Burkholderia mallei* | Glanders | Tetracycline (patients > 7 yrs) + streptomycin | Gentamicin; Chloramphenicol |
| *Burkholderia pseudomallei* | Melioidosis | Ceftazidime <u>OR</u> Chloramphenicol + sulfa + aminoglycoside for sepsis | TMP/SMX or tetracycline (patients > 7 yrs) for chronic disease |
| *Calymmatobacterium granulomatis* | Granuloma inguinale | TMP/SMX | Tetracycline (patients > 7 yrs); An aminoglycoside |

| Organism | Clinical Illness | Drug of Choice | Alternatives |
|---|---|---|---|
| *Campylobacter* spp. | Diarrhea | A macrolide | Tetracycline (patients > 7 yrs); A fluoroquinolone |
| | Sepsis, meningitis | Meropenem | An aminoglycoside |
| *Capnocytophaga canimorsus* | Sepsis following dog bite | Penicillin G | A macrolide; A 1st generation cephalosporin |
| *Capnocytophaga ochraceae* | Sepsis, abscesses | Clindamycin | A macrolide; Meropenem |
| *Chlamydia pneumoniae* (TWAR) | Pneumonia | Tetracycline | A macrolide (patients > 7 yrs) |
| *Chlamydia psittaci* | Psittacosis | Tetracycline (patients > 7 yrs) | Chloramphenicol |
| *Chlamydia trachomatis* | Lymphogranuloma venereum | Tetracycline (patients > 7 yrs) | A macrolide |
| | Urethritis, vaginitis | Tetracycline (patients > 7 yrs) or azithromycin | Erythromycin; Sulfonamide; Ampicillin |
| | Inclusion conjunctivitis of newborn | Erythromycin (oral) | Topical erythromycin, tetracycline, or sulfonamide |
| | Pneumonia in infancy | A macrolide | Ampicillin; Sulfonamide |
| | Trachoma | Topical + oral tetracycline (patients > 7 yrs) | Topical + oral sulfonamide; Azithromycin |
| *Chromobacterium violaceum* | Sepsis, pneumonia, abscesses | Chloramphenicol | Gentamicin; A fluoroquinolone |
| *Citrobacter* spp. | Meningitis, sepsis | A 3rd or 4th generation cephalosporin ± an aminoglycoside | TMP/SMX; Meropenem |

| | | | |
|---|---|---|---|
| *Clostridium* spp. | Tetanus, gas gangrene, sepsis | Metronidazole (+ antitoxin for tetanus) | Penicillin G; Clindamycin |
| *Clostridium difficile* | Antibiotic-associated colitis | Metronidazole (oral) | Vancomycin (oral) for metronidazole failures |
| *Corynebacterium diphtheriae* | Diphtheria | Erythromycin (+ antitoxin) | Penicillin G |
| *Corynebacterium*, JK group | Sepsis | Vancomycin | Penicillin G + gentamicin; A macrolide |
| *Corynebacterium minutissimum* | Erythrasma | Topical miconazole or clindamycin | A macrolide |
| *Coxiella burnetii* | Q fever | (See Rickettsia) | |
| *Cytomegalovirus* | Pneumonia, hepatitis | Ganciclovir | Foscarnet |
| *Ehrlichia chafeensis* | Human monocytic ehrlichiosis | Tetracycline (patients > 7 yrs) | Chloramphenicol |
| *Ehrlichia* (unnamed species) | Human granulocytic ehrlichiosis | Tetracycline (patients > 7 yrs) | (?) Rifampin |
| *Eikenella corrodens* | Abscesses, meningitis | Tetracycline (patients > 7 yrs); ampicillin | A macrolide; Ceftriaxone |
| *Enterobacter* spp. | Sepsis, pneumonia, wound infection | Meropenem | An aminoglycoside ± a 3rd or 4th generation cephalosporin; TMP/SMX |
| | Urinary infection | TMP/SMX | An aminoglycoside; Nitrofurantoin |
| *Enterococcus* spp. | Endocarditis, urinary infection | Ampicillin + an aminoglycoside | Vancomycin + an aminoglycoside |

NOTE: For vancomycin-resistant enterococci, consult an infectious disease expert.

| Organism | Clinical Illness | Drug of Choice | Alternatives |
|---|---|---|---|
| *Erysipelothrix rhusiopathiae* | Sepsis, cellulitis, abscesses | Ampicillin (? plus aminoglycoside) | A macrolide; A 1st generation cephalosporin |
| *Escherichia coli* | Urinary infection, not hospital acquired | A 2nd or 3rd generation cephalosporin | Ampicillin; Amoxicillin; TMP/SMX |
| | Sepsis, meningitis, pneumonia, hospital-acquired urinary infection | An aminoglycoside; A 2nd or 3rd generation cephalosporin | TMP/SMX; Meropenem |
| *Flavobacterium meningosepticum* | Sepsis, meningitis | Vancomycin plus rifampin | An aminoglycoside; TMP/SMX |
| *Francisella tularensis* | Tularemia | Gentamicin or streptomycin | Tetracycline (patients > 7 yrs); Chloramphenicol |
| *Fusobacterium* spp. | Sepsis, soft tissue infection | Penicillin G | Metronidazole; Clindamycin; Chloramphenicol |
| *Gardnerella vaginalis* | Bacterial vaginosis | Metronidazole | Clindamycin |
| *Haemophilus aphrophilus* | Sepsis, endocarditis, abscesses | Tetracycline (patients > > 7 yrs) | Ampicillin; An aminoglycoside |
| *Haemophilus ducreyi* | Chancroid | Ceftriaxone or a fluoroquinolone | A macrolide |
| *Haemophilus influenzae* | Upper respiratory infections | Augmentin®; Erythromycin-Sulfa; Azithromycin; Clarithromycin; Oral 2nd or 3rd generation cephalosporins; TMP/SMX | Amoxicillin (if beta-lactamase negative) |

| | | | |
|---|---|---|---|
| | Meningitis, arthritis, cellulitis, epiglottitis, pneumonia | Cefotaxime; Ceftriaxone | Ampicillin (if beta-lactamase negative); Chloramphenicol |
| *Helicobacter pylori* | Gastritis, peptic ulcer | Omeprazole and clarithromycin (? + amoxicillin) | Other regimens include metronidazole, tetracycline (patients > 7 yrs) |
| Herpes simplex virus | Keratoconjunctivitis | Trifluridine (topical) | Vidarabine (topical) |
| | Mucocutaneous | Acyclovir | No antimicrobial |
| | Encephalitis, disseminated disease | Acyclovir | Foscarnet |
| Human immunodeficiency virus | AIDS | Combined therapy with antiretroviral drugs | (See page 41) |
| Influenza A virus | Influenza | Amantadine; Rimantadine | (?) Ribavirin |
| *Klebsiella* spp. | Urinary tract infection | A 2nd or 3rd generation cephalosporin | TMP/SMX; Nitrofurantoin |
| | Sepsis, pneumonia, meningitis | Ceftriaxone; Cefotaxime | An aminoglycoside; TMP/SMX; Meropenem |
| *Kingella* spp. | Osteomyelitis, arthritis | Ampicillin | Other beta-lactams |
| *Legionella* spp. | Legionnaires' disease and related illnesses | A macrolide + rifampin | TMP/SMX; A fluoroquinolone |
| *Leptospira* spp. | Leptospirosis | Penicillin G | Tetracycline (patients > 7 yrs) |
| *Leptotrichia buccalis* | Vincent's angina | Penicillin G | Clindamycin; Tetracycline (patients > 7 yrs); A macrolide |

| Organism | Clinical Illness | Drug of Choice | Alternatives |
|---|---|---|---|
| *Listeria monocytogenes* | Sepsis, meningitis | Ampicillin (? plus aminoglycoside) | TMP/SMX; Vancomycin |
| *Moraxella catarrhalis* | Otitis, sinusitis, bronchitis | Augmentin®; A macrolide | TMP/SMX; A 2nd or 3rd generation cephalosporin |
| *Morganella morganii* | Urinary infection, sepsis | An aminoglycoside | A 3rd or 4th generation cephalosporin; Meropenem |
| Mycobacteria, nontuberculous (*M. kansasii, M. avium* complex) | Cervical adenitis | None (surgery) | Rifampin; Clarithromycin; Azithromycin |
| | Other diseases | Clarithromycin or azithromycin; Rifabutin; Ciprofloxacin (multiple drug therapy) | Amikacin; Clofazimine; Ethambutol |
| *Mycobacterium fortuitum* | Abscesses | An aminoglycoside + tetracycline (patients > 7 yrs) | A macrolide; Rifampin; Cefoxitin |
| *Mycobacterium leprae* | Leprosy | Dapsone + rifampin + clofazimine | Clarithromycin; Sparfloxacin; Minocycline |
| *Mycobacterium marinum* (*M. balnei*) | Papules, pustules, cold abscesses (swimmer's granuloma) | None (usually self-limited) | Clarithromycin; TMP/SMX; Tetracycline |
| *Mycobacterium tuberculosis* | Tuberculosis | Isoniazid + rifampin + pyrazinamide (? + ethambutol or streptomycin) | An aminoglycoside; Cycloserine; Ethionamide |

| | | | |
|---|---|---|---|
| *Mycoplasma hominis* | Nongonococcal urethritis | Clindamycin | Tetracycline (patients > 7 yrs) |
| *Mycoplasma pneumoniae* | Pneumonia | A macrolide | Tetracycline (patients > 7 yrs) |
| *Neisseria gonorrhoeae* | Gonorrhea | Ceftriaxone or cefixime | Spectinomycin; Penicillin G (if susceptible) |
| *Neisseria meningitidis* | Sepsis, meningitis | Penicillin G or ampicillin | A 3rd generation cephalosporin; Choloramphenicol; A sulfonamide (if susceptible) |
| *Nocardia asteroides* | Nocardiosis | TMP/SMX (+ amikacin initially) | Amikacin; Meropenem; Cycloserine; Tetracycline |
| *Pasteurella multocida* | Sepsis, abscesses | Penicillin G or ampicillin | Tetracycline (patients > 7 yrs); Augmentin® |
| *Peptostreptococcus* | Sepsis | Penicillin G or ampicillin | Clindamycin; Vancomycin |
| *Plesiomonas shigelloides* | Diarrhea, meningitis | TMP/SMX | An aminoglycoside; A 3rd generation cephalosporin |
| *Propionibacterium acnes* | Sepsis, skin lesions | Penicillin G | Tetracycline; Clindamycin; A macrolide; A 1st generation cephalosporin |
| *Proteus mirabilis* | Urinary infection, sepsis, meningitis | Ampicillin | An aminoglycoside; TMP/SMX; A cephalosporin |
| *Proteus,* other spp. | Urinary infection, sepsis, meningitis | Cefotaxime; Ceftriaxone | Meropenem; An aminoglycoside |
| *Providencia* spp. | Sepsis | Cefotaxime; Ceftriaxone | TMP/SMX; Meropenem; An aminoglycoside |

| Organism | Clinical Illness | Drug of Choice | Alternatives |
|---|---|---|---|
| *Pseudomonas aeruginosa* | Urinary infection | Anti-*Pseudomonas* beta-lactam | An aminoglycoside |
| | Sepsis, pneumonia | Anti-*Pseudomonas* beta-lactam + an aminoglycoside | Ciprofloxacin |
| *Pseudomonas cepacia* | See *Burkholderia* | | |
| *Pseudomonas mallei* | See *Burkholderia* | | |
| *Pseudomonas pseudomallei* | See *Burkholderia* | | |
| Respiratory syncytial virus | Bronchiolitis, pneumonia | Ribavirin | None |
| *Rhodococcus equi* | Necrotizing pneumonia | Vancomycin (? + a fluoroquinolone) | An aminoglycoside; A macrolide; Rifampin |
| *Rickettsia* | Rocky Mountain spotted fever, Q fever, typhus, rickettsialpox | Tetracycline (patients > 7 yrs) | Chloramphenicol; A fluoroquinolone |
| *Rochalimaea henselae* | See *Bartonella* | | |
| *Salmonella* spp. | Focal infections, typhoid fever, sepsis | Ceftriaxone; Cefotaxime; A fluoroquinolone | TMP/SMX; Chloramphenicol; Ampicillin (if susceptible) |
| *Serratia marcescens* | Sepsis, pneumonia | Ceftriaxone; Cefotaxime | TMP/SMX; An aminoglycoside; Meropenem |
| *Shigella* spp. | Enteritis, urinary infection, vaginitis | Cefixime | A fluoroquinolone; TMP/SMX; Ampicillin; Ceftriaxone |

| | | | |
|---|---|---|---|
| *Spirillum minus* | Rat-bite fever (sodoku) | Penicillin G or ampicillin | Tetracycline (patients > 7 yrs); An aminoglycoside |
| *Staphylococcus aureus* | Skin infections | A 1st generation cephalosporin | Cloxacillin; A macrolide |
| | Pneumonia, sepsis, osteomyelitis, etc. | Oxacillin or nafcillin; A 1st generation cephalosporin | Vancomycin; Clindamycin |
| *Staphylococcus*, coagulase negative | Sepsis, infected CNS shunts, urinary infection | Vancomycin | If susceptible: nafcillin (or related drug); (?) TMP/SMX |
| *Staphylococcus* spp., methicillin-resistant | Sepsis, focal infections | Vancomycin (? + rifampin and/or gentamicin) | TMP/SMX; A fluoroquinolone |
| *Stenotrophomonas maltophilia* | Sepsis | TMP/SMX | Ceftazidime; Ticarcillin-clavulanate |
| *Streptobacillus moniliformis* | Rat-bite fever (Haverhill fever) | Penicillin G or ampicillin | Tetracycline (patients > 7 yrs); An aminoglycoside |
| *Streptococcus*, Groups A, B, C, and G, anaerobic | Pharyngitis, impetigo, adenitis | Penicillin V or amoxicillin; Benzathine penicillin | A macrolide; A 1st generation cephalosporin; Clindamycin |
| | Pneumonia, sepsis, meningitis | Penicillin G or ampicillin | A 1st generation cephalosporin; Vancomycin |
| *Streptococcus*, viridans group | Endocarditis | Penicillin G + gentamicin | Vancomycin; A 3rd generation cephalosporin |
| *Streptococcus pneumoniae* | Pneumonia, otitis, sinusitis | Penicillin V or G; Amoxicillin | A macrolide; A cephalosporin |
| | Meningitis, arthritis, sepsis | Penicillin G | Vancomycin (for penicillin-resistant strains); Cefotaxime or ceftriaxone for relatively resistant strains |

| Organism | Clinical Illness | Drug of Choice | Alternatives |
|---|---|---|---|
| *Treponema pallidum* | Syphilis | Penicillin G | Tetracycline (patients > 7 yrs); Ceftriaxone |
| *Treponema pertenue* | Yaws | Penicillin G | Tetracycline (patients > 7 yrs) |
| *Ureaplasma urealyticum* | Genitourinary infections | A macrolide | Tetracycline (patients > 7 yrs) |
| Varicella-zoster virus | Disseminated disease, zoster (shingles) | Acyclovir | Vidarabine; Foscarnet |
| *Vibrio cholerae* | Cholera | Tetracycline (patients > 7 yrs) | TMP/SMX; A fluoroquinolone |
| *Vibrio vulnificus* | Sepsis | Tetracycline (patients > 7 yrs) | A 3rd generation cephalosporin |
| *Yersinia enterocolitica* | Enteritis, arthritis, sepsis | (?) Tetracycline (patients > 7 yrs); TMP/SMX | A macrolide; An aminoglycoside; A 3rd generation cephalosporin |
| *Yersinia pestis* | Plague | Streptomycin + chlor-amphenicol or tetra-cycline (patients > 7 yrs) | Other aminoglycoside |
| *Yersinia pseudotuberculosis* | Adenitis | (?) Tetracycline; (?) TMP/SMX | An aminoglycoside; A 3rd generation cephalosporin; A fluoroquinolone |

# VI. ANTIFUNGAL THERAPY

| Infection | Therapy | Comments |
|---|---|---|
| SYSTEMIC INFECTIONS | | |
| **Aspergillosis** | Amphotericin B 1.0 mg/kg IV daily as 3–4-hour infusion in 5% dextrose solution (no saline); Total dosage 30–35 mg/kg given over period of 6 wks or longer; For patients with renal failure and those not tolerating or failing to respond, Abelcet® 5 mg/kg IV, or AmBisome® 3–5 mg/kg or Amphotec 3–5 mg/kg daily can be used; Itraconazole may be considered for indolent, non-CNS disease | Treat for tissue invasion, not colonization; Monitor K, Mg, $HCO_3$, Hgb, and renal function; Azotemia common; Sodium loading may help azotemia; Total dosage and duration of therapy individualized (For allergic bronchopulmonary aspergillosis, see page 27) |
| **Blastomycosis** (North American) | Itraconazole 200–400 mg/day (adults), (?) 4 mg/kg/day (pediatric dosage not established) PO OR amphotericin B (as above) for severe disease; × 6 mos | Alternative: ketoconazole 6 mg/kg/day PO div q12–24h |
| **Candidiasis** | | |
| - Disseminated infection | Amphotericin B (as above) but daily dosage 0.5–0.75 mg/kg OR amphotericin B PLUS flucytosine 100 mg/kg/day PO div q6h; OR Abelcet, AmBisome® or Amphotec® (as above); Fluconazole 6–12 mg/kg IV or PO daily for noncompromized host (some strains resistant to fluconazole) | Hematologic toxicity and diarrhea with flucytosine; Keep serum concentration < 100 µg/ml; Replace IV catheter in catheter-associated candidemia |
| - Urinary infection | Fluconazole 3–6 mg/kg once daily OR flucytosine 50 mg/kg/day div q6h; Amphotericin B (50 µg/ml) bladder irrigation if catheter in place | Stopping antibiotic or removing Foley catheter sometimes leads to spontaneous cure in the normal host |

| | | |
|---|---|---|
| - Oropharyngeal, esophageal | Clotrimazole 10 mg troche PO five times daily × 7 days OR fluconazole 3–6 mg/kg once daily OR itraconazole oral solution 10–20 ml (adult dose) swished in mouth and swallowed once daily OR amphotericin B suspension 1 ml q.i.d. | Amphotericin B IV for severe disease or febrile neutropenic patients; Miconazole gel (not available in United States) best for thrush in infants |
| **Chromomycosis** | Flucytosine OR itraconazole (as above) | |
| **Coccidioidomycosis** | Amphotericin B (as above) for severe, non-CNS disease OR (for non–life-threatening disease) itraconazole 200 mg bid PO (adult dose) OR fluconazole 6–12 mg/kg once daily for meningitis | Consider intrathecal amphotericin B fluconazole failures in meningitis |
| **Cryptococcosis** | Amphotericin B 0.7 mg/kg IV daily ± flucytosine 100 mg/kg/day PO div q6h; Monitor flucytosine serum concentrations | For HIV-positive, amphotericin B × 2 wks, then fluconazole 6–12 mg/kg once daily for 10 wks, then 4 mg/kg daily indefinitely |
| **Histoplasmosis** | Amphotericin B 0.5 mg/kg IV daily OR (for non–life-threatening disease) itraconazole 200 mg b.i.d. PO (adults) | Ketoconazole (as above) as alternative |
| **Mucormycosis** (zygomycosis) | Amphotericin B (as for aspergillosis) × 6 wks or longer | Surgery, as necessary; Control of diabetes mellitus, if present |
| **Paracoccidioidomycosis** | Itraconazole 100 mg/day PO (adults) OR amphotericin B 0.5 mg/kg IV daily or longer | Ketoconazole (as above) as alternative; Sulfa drugs less effective but inexpensive |
| **Phaeohyphomycosis** | Amphotericin B (as for aspergillosis) × 3 wks or longer | Surgery, as necessary; Itraconazole (as above) for indolent, non-CNS disease may be useful |

| Infection | Therapy | Comments |
|---|---|---|
| ***Pneumocystis carinii* pneumonia** | Trimethoprim-sulfamethoxazole 15–20 mg <u>OR</u> pentamidine isethionate 4 mg base/kg/day IV daily × 10–14 days; Alternatives: trimethoprim and dapsone; primaquine and clindamycin; trimetrexate and folinic acid; atovaquone for nonsevere disease | Prophylaxis: 5 mg TMP, 25 daily or three times weekly <u>OR</u> dapsone 1 mg/kg PO once daily |
| ***Pseudallescheria boydii* and *Scedosporium apiospermum* infection** | Miconazole 20–40 mg/kg/day IV div q8h × 3 wks or longer | Ketoconazole or itraconazole may be effective |
| **Sporotrichosis** | Itraconazole 100–200 mg/day PO (adult dosage); amphotericin B (as for aspergillosis) or itraconazole 200 mg b.i.d. for extracutaneous disease | Alternative: Saturated solution of potassium iodide 1–2 drops per year of age, three times daily PO (maximum 30 drops t.i.d.) until lymphocutaneous lesions resolved (give with fruit juice or milk) |
| <u>LOCALIZED MUCOCUTANEOUS INFECTIONS</u> | | |
| **Dermatophytoses** | | |
| - Scalp (tinea capitis, including kerion); *Trichophyton*, *microsporum*, *Epidermophyton*, spp. | Griseofulvin ultramicrosized 10 mg/kg or microsized 15 mg/kg once daily × 1–2 mos or longer (taken with milk or fatty foods to augment absorption) <u>OR</u> ketoconazole 6 mg/kg/day div q12–24h; Itraconazole or terbinafine may be useful | Topical antifungal agent may prevent recurrence from endothrix spores; Selenium sulfide shampoo twice weekly may be useful adjunct |
| - Glabrous skin, hands or feet | Topical butenafine, ciclopirox, clotrimazole, econazole, ketoconazole, miconazole, naftifine, sulconazole, terbinafine, and tolnaftate equally effective; Apply twice daily × 7–10 days | Undecylemic acid less effective; Longer treatment needed for palmar/plantar infection; Keep toe webs and groin dry; Treat bacterial superinfection |

| | | |
|---|---|---|
| - Tinea versicolor [*Pityrosporum ovale* (*Malassezia furfur*)] | Selenium sulfide (Selsun) OR topical clotrimazole (or related drug) applied twice daily × 7–10 days | Recurrence common; Itraconazole useful for extensive lesions |
| - Tinea unguium (onychomycosis) | Itraconazole 200 mg bid PO or terbinafine 500 mg daily (adult doses) for [illegible] wk per mo × 3 mos (hands) or 6 mos (toes) until new nail growth | Recurrence or partial response common |
| **Candidiasis** | | |
| - Benign mucocutaneous | Topical imidazole derivative (e.g., clotrimazole, econazole, miconazole, oxiconazole) three to four times daily × 7–10 days | 0.5% aqueous gentian violet for refractory cases |
| - Oropharyngeal, esophageal | (See Disseminated infection, above) | |
| - Chronic mucocutaneous | Itraconazole 200 mg PO daily (adult dosage) OR fluconazole 3 mg/kg daily PO until lesions clear | Occurs in hosts with variety of immune defects |
| - Vulvovaginal | Vaginal cream with butoconazole, clotrimazole, miconazole, terconazole, or tioconazole; OR vaginal tablets/suppositories of clotrimazole, miconazole, terconazole; all at bedtime × 3–7 days; OR (for adult) 150-mg dose of fluconazole × 1 day | Avoid fluconazole in pregnancy |

# VII. ANTIPARASITIC THERAPY

NOTE: Familiarize yourself with the toxic potentials of these drugs and monitor the patient accordingly. For some of the parasitic diseases, the preferred therapy is use of drugs available only from the Centers for Disease Control; these drugs are indicated by "(CDC)." Consultation for diagnostic tests and detailed information about experimental drugs are available from the CDC; they will send drugs to you. The telephone number is 1-770-488-7788.

| Disease/Organism | Treatment |
|---|---|
| **AMEBIASIS**<br>*Entamoeba histolytica* | |
| - Asymptomatic carrier | Iodoquinol (formerly diiodohydroxyquin) 30–40 mg/kg/day (max 2 g) PO div q8h × 20 days OR paromomycin 30 mg/kg/day PO div q8h × 7–10 days OR diloxanide furoate (CDC) 20 mg/kg/day PO div q8h × 10 days |
| - Mild to moderate colitis | Metronidazole 35–50 mg/kg/day PO div q8h × 10 days OR tinidazole (not available in United States) 50 mg/kg/day PO (max 2 g) × 3 days FOLLOWED BY iodoquinol or paromomycin PO, as above, × 20 days to eliminate cysts |
| - Severe colitis, liver abscess | Metronidazole 35–50 mg/kg/day PO, IV div q8h × 10 days FOLLOWED BY iodoquinol or paromomycin, as above |
| **AMEBIC MENINGOENCEPHALITIS**<br>*Naegleria* spp., *Acanthamoeba* spp., *Hartmannella* spp. | Amphotericin B 1 mg/kg/day IV × (?) 3–4 wks, (?) PLUS miconazole and rifampin for *Naegleria*; Intrathecal miconazole (10 mg) daily may be helpful; *Acanthamoeba* susceptible *in vitro* to ketoconazole, flucytosine, pentamidine |
| *Ancylostoma caninum* | See EOSINOPHILIC COLITIS |
| *Ancylostoma duodenale* | See HOOKWORM |
| **ANGIOSTRONGYLIASIS**<br>*Angiostrongylus* spp. | Mebendazole 100 mg PO b.i.d. × 5 days for *A. cantonensis*; Thiabendazole 50–75 mg/kg/day (max 3 g) PO div q8h for × 3 days OR mebendazole 200–400 mg PO t.i.d. × 10 days for *A. costaricensis* |

| Infection | Treatment |
|---|---|
| **ANISAKIASIS**<br>*Anasakis* spp. | Removal by fibroendoscopy or surgery |
| **ASCARIASIS**<br>*Ascaris lumbricoides* | Mebendazole 100 mg PO b.i.d. × 3 days (alternative, 500 mg once) <u>OR</u> albendazole 400 mg PO, one dose <u>OR</u> pyrantel pamoate 11 mg/kg (max 1 g) PO, one dose |
| **BABESIOSIS**<br>*Babesia* spp. | Clindamycin 30 mg/kg/day PO div q8h <u>PLUS</u> quinine 25 mg/kg/day PO div q8h × 7 days effective in limited experience; Exchange blood transfusion reported helpful; Atovaquone plus azithromycin may be effective |
| **BALANTIDIASIS**<br>*Balantidium coli* | Metronidazole 35–50 mg/kg/day PO div q8h × 5 days <u>OR</u> tetracycline (patient > 7 yrs) 40 mg/kg/day PO div q6h × 10 days <u>OR</u> iodoquinol 40 mg/kg/day (max 2 g/day) PO div q8h × 20 days |
| **BLASTOCYSTIASIS**<br>*Blastocystis hominis* | Metronidazole 35–50 mg/kg/day PO div q8h × 10 days <u>OR</u> iodoquinol 40 mg/kg/day (max 2 g) PO div q8h × 20 days (Need for treatment in normal hosts is controversial) |
| **CAPILLARIASIS**<br>*Capillaria philippinensis* | Mebendazole 200 mg PO twice daily × 20 days <u>OR</u> albendazole 400 mg PO daily × 10 days |
| **CHAGAS' DISEASE**<br>*Trypanosoma cruzi* | See TRYPANOSOMIASIS |
| *Clonorchis sinensis* | See FLUKES |
| **CRYPTOSPORIDIOSIS**<br>*Cryptosporidium parvum* | No proven effective therapy; Paromomycin or azithromycin may be effective |
| **CUTANEOUS LARVA MIGRANS** or **CREEPING ERUPTION**<br>(Cutaneous hookworm) | Thiabendazole suspension topically b.i.d. × 2–5 days <u>OR</u> ivermectin 200 μg/kg PO, once <u>OR</u> albendazole 400 mg once daily PO × 3 days <u>OR</u> thiabendazole 50 mg/kg/day (max 3 g) PO div q12h × 3 days; <u>NOTE</u>: Ethylene chloride spray and carbon dioxide snow are effective but painful and sometimes damage tissue |

| Disease/Organism | Treatment |
|---|---|
| **CYCLOSPORIASIS**<br>*Cyclospora* sp.<br>(Cyanobacterium-like agent) | Trimethoprim-sulfamethoxazole (10 mg TMP–50 mg SMX/kg/day) PO div q12h × 5–7 days |
| **CYSTICERCOSIS**<br>*Cysticercus cellulosae* | Albendazole 15 mg/kg/day PO div q12h (max 800 mg/day) × 8–30 days OR praziquantel 50 mg/kg/day PO div q8h × 15 days; For CNS cysticercosis with multiple lesions give steroids before first dose (Steroids and Dilantin can affect metabolism of albendazole and praziquantel; Therapy for active lesions only; Surgery when indicated) |
| **DIENTAMEBIASIS**<br>*Dientamoeba fragilis* | Iodoquinol 40 mg/kg/day (max 2 g) PO div q8h × 20 days OR tetracycline (patients > 7 yrs) 40 mg/kg/day PO div q6h × 7–10 days OR paromomycin 25 mg/kg/day PO div q8h × 7 days |
| *Diphyllobothrium latum* | See TAPEWORMS |
| **DIROFILARIASIS**<br>*Dirofilaria immitis* | Surgical excision of subcutaneous or pulmonary nodules; Albendazole possibly effective |
| **DRACUNCULIASIS**<br>*Dracunculus medinensis*<br>(Guinea worm) | Metronidazole 25 mg/kg/day PO div q8h × 10 days (not curative but reduces inflammation); IN ADDITION remove worm by winding out a few cm each day |
| **ECHINOCOCCOSIS**<br>*Echinococcus granulosus* | Surgical treatment when indicated; Albendazole 15 mg/kg/day PO div q12h × 28 days followed by 14 days without drug; give two or three cycles of therapy, if necessary |
| *Entamoeba histolytica* | See AMEBIASIS |
| *Enterobius vermicularis* | See PINWORMS |
| *Fasciola hepatica* | See FLUKES |
| **EOSINOPHILIC COLITIS**<br>*Ancylostoma caninum* | Mebendazole 100 mg PO b.i.d. × 3 days OR albendazole 400 mg PO once |

| | |
|---|---|
| **EOSINOPHILIC MENINGITIS** | See ANGIOSTRONGYLIASIS and GNATHOSTOMIASIS |
| **FILARIASIS** | |
| - River blindness<br>*Onchocerca volvulus* | Ivermectin 150 μg/kg PO, one dose; Repeat q6–12mos; Antihistamines or corticosteroids for allergic reactions |
| - Other forms (loa loa, tropical eosinophilia) *Wuchereria bancrofti*, *Brugia malayi* | Diethylcarbamazine 1 mg/kg PO on day 1, 1 mg/kg t.i.d. on day 2, 2 mg/kg t.i.d. on day 3; then 6 mg/kg/day (9 mg/kg/day for loa loa) PO div q8h × 18 days; Antihistamines or corticosteroids for allergic reactions; Surgical excision of subcutaneous nodules, preferably before drug therapy; Ivermectin may be effective; <u>NOTE</u>: In heavy infections consider giving albendazole or ivermectin initially to reduce counts before diethylcarbamazine therapy in loa loa |
| **FLUKES** | |
| - Sheep liver fluke (*Fasciola hepatica*)<br>- Lung fluke (*Paragonimus westermani*)<br>- Chinese liver fluke (*Clonorchis sinensis*) and others (*Fasciolopsis*, *Heterophyes*, *Metagonimus*, *Opisthorchis*) | Praziquantel 75 mg/kg PO div q8h × 1 day × 2 days for *P. westermani*) is the drug of choice for all fluke infections except *F. hepatica* for which bithionol (CDC) is given (30–50 mg/kg PO div q.i.d. on alternate days × 10–15 doses) |
| **GIARDIASIS**<br>*Giardia lamblia* | Furazolidone 6–8 mg/kg/day PO div q6h × 7–10 days <u>OR</u> metronidazole 15 mg/kg/day PO div q8h × 5 days; Quinacrine effective but not easily available in the United States (All can have Antabuse-like effect) |
| **GNATHOSTOMIASIS**<br>*Gnathostoma spinigerum* | Surgical removal <u>PLUS</u> albendazole 15 mg/kg/day PO div q12h × 21 days; Ivermectin may be effective |
| **HOOKWORM**<br>*Necator americanus*, *Ancylostoma duodenale* | Mebendazole 100 mg PO b.i.d. × 3 days (alternative, 500 mg once) <u>OR</u> pyrantel pamoate 11 mg/kg (max 1 g/day) PO daily × 3 days; <u>OR</u> albendazole 10 mg/kg (max 400 mg), once (repeat dosing of albendazole sometimes necessary) |

| Disease/Organism | Treatment |
|---|---|
| *Hymenolepis nana* | See TAPEWORMS |
| **ISOSPORIASIS**<br>*Isospora belli* | Trimethoprim-sulfamethoxazole 10 mg TMP–50 mg SMX/kg/day PO div q6h × 10 days; Then, 5 mg TMP–25 mg SMX/kg/day PO div q12h × 3 wks; Pyrimethamine may be effective |
| **LEISHMANIASIS, including kala azar**<br>*Leishmania braziliensis*, *L. donovani*, *L. tropica*, *L. mexicana* | Stibogluconate sodium (CDC) 20 mg/kg/day (max 800 mg) IM or IV, daily × 20–28 days; ALTERNATIVES, pentamidine isethionate 2–4 mg/kg/day IM daily for 14 days OR amphotericin B 0.5–1 mg/kg/day IV × 4–8 wks |
| **LICE**<br>*Pediculus capitis* or *humanus*, *Pthirus pubis* | Permethrin 1% (Nix Creme Rinse) OR pyrethins (RID, A-200 Pyrinate liquid or shampoo, R&C Shampoo) OR lindane (Kwell) applied topically once (follow manufacturer's instructions for use); Repeat in 1 wk; OR ivermectin 200 mcg/kg PO, one dose; For eyelash infestation, use petrolatum; Launder bedding and clothing; For head lice, remove nits with comb designed for that purpose |
| **MALARIA** | CDC Malaria Hotline 1-770-488-7788 and online information at www.cdc.gov; It is advisable for physicians who are not familiar with treating malaria to consult with CDC physicians; The following suggestions for treatment do not cover all situations |
| **Prophylaxis** | |
| - For areas without chloroquine-resistant *Plasmodium falciparum* | Chloroquine 5 mg base/kg (max 300 mg) PO once weekly, beginning 1 wk before arrival in malarial zone and continuing for 4 wks after last exposure (drugs available in liquid form outside the United States); PLUS (optional) beginning with final 2 wks of chloroquine Rx, primaquine 0.3 mg base/kg PO daily × 14 days after departure from endemic area for individuals heavily exposed to mosquitoes |
| - For areas where chloroquine-resistant *P. falciparum* exists | Mefloquine for children > 45 kg 250 mg PO once weekly starting 1 wk before travel and for 4 wks after leaving area; for children 5–9 kg, ⅛ tab; 10–19 kg, ¼ tab; 20–30 kg, ½ tab; 31–45 kg, ¾ tab OR doxycycline (patient > 7 yrs) 2 mg/kg (max 100 mg) PO daily |

| Treatment of disease | |
|---|---|
| - *Plasmodium vivax*, *P. ovale*, *P. malariae*, chloroquine-susceptible *P. falciparum* | Chloroquine 10 mg base/kg (max 600 mg) PO stat, then 5 mg base/kg at 6 hrs, 24 hrs and 48 hrs after initial dose (alternative: at 6, 12, 24, and 36 hrs); For parenteral therapy, quinidine 10 mg/kg (max 600 mg) IV (1-hr infusion) followed by continuous infusion of 0.02 mg/kg/min until oral therapy can be given (3 days max); It is advisable to monitor patients receiving quinidine in an ICU setting; Prevention of relapse (*P. vivax*, *P. ovale*): primaquine 0.3 mg base/kg/day × 14 days |
| - *P. falciparum* chloroquine-resistant | Quinine 25 mg/kg/day (max 2 g/day) PO div q8h × 3 days (or longer) AND doxycycline (patients > 7 yrs) 2 mg/kg daily × 7 OR Fansidar (pyrimethamine-sulfadoxine): < 1 yr, ¼ tab; 1–3 yrs, ½ tab; 4–8 yrs, 1 tab; 9–14 yrs, 2 tab; > 14 yrs, 3 tabs as a single dose on last day of quinine; NOTE: Several alternative regimens have been reported for Fansidar-resistant infections: Check with the CDC; For parenteral therapy, quinidine, as above; NOTE: Corticosteroids are contraindicated in cerebral malaria; Iron chelation therapy may be beneficial in cerebral malaria |
| *Paragonimus westermani* | See FLUKES |
| **MICROSPORIDIOSIS**<br>*Encephalitozoon* sp., *Enterocytozoon* sp., *Vittaforma* sp. | Albendazole 400 mg PO b.i.d. (adult dosage) |
| **PINWORMS**<br>*Enterobius vermicularis* | Mebendazole 100 mg PO, one dose OR albendazole 400 mg PO, one dose OR pyrantel pamoate 11 mg/kg (max 1 gm) PO, one dose; Repeat treatment in 2 wks |
| **PNEUMOCYSTIS PNEUMONIA**<br>*Pneumocystis carinii* | See page 58 |
| **SCABIES**<br>*Sarcoptes scabei* | Permethrim 5% cream applied to entire body (including scalp in infants), left on for 8–14 hr before bathing OR lindane (Kwell) lotion applied to all of body below neck, leave on overnight, bathe in a.m. OR ivermectin 200 µg/kg PO, one dose; Launder bedding and clothing; Topical corticosteroid after treatment for severe, persistent itching |

| Disease/Organism | Treatment |
|---|---|
| **SCHISTOSOMIASIS** *Schistosoma haematobium, S. japonicum, S. mansoni, S. mekongi* | Praziquantel 40 (for *S. haematobium* and *S. mansoni*) –60 (for *S. japonicum* and *S. mekongi*) mg/kg PO in 2–3 doses taken in 1 day |
| **STRONGYLOIDIASIS** *Strongyloides stercoralis* | Invermectin 200 µg/kg PO daily × 2 days OR thiabendazole 50 mg/kg/day (max 3 g/day) PO div q12h × 2 days (5 days or longer for disseminated disease) |
| **TAPEWORMS** | |
| - *Cysticercus cellulosae* | See CYSTICERCOSIS |
| - *Echinococcus granulosus* | See ECHINOCOCCOSIS |
| - *Taenia saginata, T. solium, Hymenolepis nana, Diphyllobothrium latum, Dipylidium caninum* | Praziquantel 5–10 mg/kg PO × 1 dose (25 mg/kg for *H. nana*) OR niclosamide tablet (not available in the United States) approximately 40 mg/kg PO chewed thoroughly × 1 dose |
| **TOXOPLASMOSIS** *Toxoplasma gondii* | Pyrimethamine 2 mg/kg/day PO div q12h × 3 days (max 100 mg) then 1 mg/kg/day (max 25 mg every day) PO (supplemental folinic acid) AND sulfadiazine 120 mg/kg/day PO div q6h (max 6 g/day): For prophylaxis in pregnancy, spiramycin (CDC) 50–100 mg/kg/day PO div q6h; Treatment continued for 4 wks after resolution of illness (See page 8 for congenital toxoplasmosis); Corticosteroids given for ocular infection; Prophylaxis: trimethoprim-sulfamethoxazole, as for *Pneumocystis* (page 60) |
| **TRICHINOSIS** *Trichinella spiralis* | Anti-inflammatory drugs; Steroids for CNS or severe symptoms; Mebendazole 200–400 mg PO t.i.d. × 3 days, then 400–500 mg t.i.d. × 10 days |
| **TRICHOMONIASIS** *Trichomonas vaginalis* | Metronidazole 40 mg/kg (max 2 g) PO × 1 dose OR metronidazole 15 mg/kg/day (max 1 g/day) PO div q8h × 7 days; Treat sex partners |

| | |
|---|---|
| **TRICHOSTRONGYLIASIS**<br>*Trichostrongylus orientalis* | Mebendazole 100 mg PO b.i.d. × 3 days OR pyrantel pamoate 11 mg/kg, one dose OR albendazole 400 mg PO once |
| *Trichuris trichiura* | See WHIPWORM |
| **TRYPANOSOMIASIS** | |
| - **CHAGAS' DISEASE**<br>*Trypanosoma cruzi* | Nifurtimox (CDC) or benznidazole (CDC); Obtain drug and dosage recommendations from CDC; Gamma interferon has been added to regimen in some patients |
| - **SLEEPING SICKNESS**<br>*T. brucei gambiense*; *T. brucei rhodesiense* | Acute stage: suramin (CDC) 20 mg/kg (max 1 g) IV on days 1, 3, 7, 14, and 21 OR pentamidine isethionate 4 mg/kg/day IM × 10 days<br>Late disease with CNS involvement: Melarsoprol (CDC) initial dose 0.36 mg/kg IV, gradually increase dosage to maximum dose of 3.6 mg/kg given at 1- to 5-day intervals for total of 10 doses (18–25 mg/kg) during a 1-mo period<br>For acute and CNS disease: eflornithine (available from WHO) IV div q6h × 14 days, 400 mg/kg/day followed by 300 mg/kg/day PO × 3–4 wks |
| **VISCERAL LARVA MIGRANS**<br>*Toxocara canis*; *T. cati* | Albendazole 400 mg PO b.i.d. × 3–5 days OR diethylcarbamazine 6 mg/kg/day PO div q8h × 7–10 days OR mebendazole 100–200 mg PO b.i.d. × 5 days; Corticosteroids for severe symptoms and for eye involvement |
| **WHIPWORM (TRICHURIASIS)**<br>*Trichuris trichiura* | Mebendazole 100 mg PO b.i.d. × 3 days OR albendazole 400 mg PO, one dose |
| *Wuchereria bancrofti* | See FILARIASIS |

# VIII. ALPHABETICAL LISTING OF ANTIBIOTICS WITH DOSAGE FORMS AND USUAL DOSAGES

NOTES:
1. When a range of dosage is given, the higher dosages are generally indicated for serious illnesses.
2. In some cases the dosages indicated differ from the manufacturers' recommendations in the package inserts.
3. IV preparations available in ready-to-use "piggy-back" bottles are not included in the tabulated dosage forms.

| Generic and Trade Names | Dosage Form | Route | Dosage | Interval |
|---|---|---|---|---|
| Acyclovir<br>Zovirax®, generic | 500-, 1000-mg vial | IV | 25–50 mg/kg/day | q8h |
| | 200 mg/5 ml susp | PO | 80 mg/kg/day | q6h |
| | 200-mg cap; 400-, 800-mg tab | PO | 1 cap five times daily; 1 tab four times daily (adults) | |
| Albendazole<br>Albenza® | 200-mg tab | PO | 15 mg/kg/day | q12h |
| Amantadine HCl<br>Symmetrel®, generic | 100-mg cap<br>50 mg/5 ml syrup | PO | 5–8 mg/kg/day<br>(max 200 mg/day) | q12h |
| Amikacin sulfate | 0.5-, 1-g vial | IM, IV | 15–22.5 mg/kg/day (see page 4 regarding q24h dosing) | q8h |
| Amoxicillin trihydrate<br>Amoxil®, Trimox®,<br>Wymox®, generic | 250-, 500-mg cap<br>500-, 875-mg tab<br>125, 250 mg/5-ml susp<br>125-, 250-mg chewable tab<br>50 mg/1 ml drops | PO | 40 mg/kg/day | q8h |

| | | | | |
|---|---|---|---|---|
| Amoxicillin and clavulanate potassium<br>Augmentin® | 7:1 Formulation:<br>875/125-mg tab<br>200/28.5-, 400/57-mg chewable tab<br>200/28.5, 400/57 mg/5 ml susp | PO | 7:1 Formulation:<br>45-mg amoxicillin component/kg/day | q12h |
| | 4:1 Formulation:<br>500/125-mg tab<br>125/31.25-, 250/62.5-mg chewable tab<br>125/31.25, 250/62.5 mg/5 ml susp | | 4:1 Formulation:<br>30-mg amoxicillin component/kg/day | q8h |
| Amphotericin B<br>Fungizone® | 50-mg vial | IV | 0.25–1 mg/kg/day | q1–2 days |
| | 100 mg/ml susp | PO | 4–12 ml/day | q6h |
| Amphotericin B, cholesteryl sulfate<br>AMPHOTEC® | 50-, 100-mg vial | IV | 3–5 mg/kg/day | q24h |
| Amphotericin B, lipid complex<br>ABELCET® | 100-mg vial | IV | 5 mg/kg/day | q24h |
| Amphotericin B, liposomal<br>AmBisome® | 50-mg vial | IV | 3–5 mg/kg/day | q24h |
| Ampicillin and Ampicillin trihydrate<br>Omnipen®, Principen® generic | 250-, 500-mg cap<br>125, 250/5 ml susp<br>100 mg/ml drops | PO | 50 mg/kg/day | q6h |

| Generic and Trade Names | Dosage Form | Route | Dosage | Interval |
|---|---|---|---|---|
| Ampicillin, sodium<br>Omnipen®, generic | 0.125-, 0.25-, 0.5-, 1-, 2-, 4-g vials | IM, IV | 100–200 mg/kg/day<br>(meningitis 200–400) | q6h |
| Ampicillin/Sulbactam<br>Unasyn® | 1 g amp/0.5 g sul, 2 g amp/1 g sul | IV | As per ampicillin; Not approved for infants < 1 yr | q6h |
| Amprenavir<br>Agenerase® | 50-, 150-mg cap<br>75 mg/5 ml oral solution | PO | 1200 mg b.i.d.<br>(adult dosage) | q12h |
| Atovaquone<br>Mepron® | 750 mg/5 ml susp | PO | (?) 40 mg/kg/day with meals | q8h |
| Azithromycin<br>Zithromax® | 250-mg cap<br>600-mg tab<br>100, 200 mg/5 ml susp | PO | Otitis/pneumonia: 10 mg/kg/day loading dose, then 5 mg/kg/day<br>Pharyngitis: 12 mg/kg/day | q24h |
| | 500-mg vial | IV | | |
| Aztreonam<br>Azactam® | 0.5-, 1-, 2-g vial | IM, IV | 90–120 mg/kg/day | q6–8h |
| Bacampicillin Hcl<br>Spectrobid® | 400-mg tab (equivalent to 280 mg ampicillin)<br>125 mg/5 ml | PO | 25–50 mg/kg/day | q12h |
| Carbenicillin indanyl sodium<br>Geocillin® | 382-mg tab | PO | 30–50 mg/kg/day | q6h |
| Cefaclor<br>Ceclor®, generic | 125, 187, 250, 375 mg/5 ml susp<br>250-, 500-mg cap | PO | 40 mg/kg/day | q8–12h |

| | | | | |
|---|---|---|---|---|
| Cefadroxil monohydrate<br>Duricef® | 500-mg cap, 1-g tab<br>125, 250, 500 mg/5 ml susp | PO | 30 mg/kg/day | q12–24h |
| Cefamandole nafate<br>Mandol® | 0.5-, 1-, 2-g vial | IV, IM | 100–150 mg/kg/day | q4–6h |
| Cefazolin sodium<br>Ancef®, Kefzol® | 0.5-, 1-g vial | IM, IV | 50–100 mg/kg/day | q8h |
| Cefdinir<br>Omnicef® | 300-mg cap<br>125 mg/5 ml solution | PO | 14 mg/kg/day | q12–24h |
| Cefepime HCl<br>Maxipime® | 1-, 2-g vial | IV, IM | 1–4 q/day for adults<br>(Not approved for children) | q12h |
| Cefixime<br>Suprax® | 200-, 400-mg tab<br>100 mg/5 ml susp | PO | 8 mg/kg/day | q12–24h |
| Cefonicid sodium<br>Monocid® | 1-g vial | IV, IM | (?) 20–40 mg/kg/day<br>(Not approved for children) | q24h |
| Cefoperazone sodium<br>Cefobid® | 1-, 2-g vial | IV, IM | 100–150 mg/kg/day<br>(Not approved for children) | q8–12h |
| Cefotaxime sodium<br>Claforan® | 0.5-, 1-, 2-g vial | IV, IM | 50–180 mg/kg/day<br>(meningitis 300 div q6h) | q6–8h |
| Cefotetan disodium<br>Cefotan® | 1-, 2-g vial | IV, IM | (?) 40–80 mg/kg/day<br>(Not approved for children) | q12h |
| Cefoxitin sodium<br>Mefoxin® | 1-, 2-g vial | IV, IM | 80–160 mg/kg/day | q4–6h |

| Generic and Trade Names | Dosage Form | Route | Dosage | Interval |
| --- | --- | --- | --- | --- |
| Cefpodoxime proxetil<br>Vantin® | 100-, 200-mg tab<br>50, 100 mg/5 ml susp | PO | 10 mg/kg/day<br>(max 400 mg) | q12–24h |
| Cefprozil<br>Cefzil® | 250-, 500-mg tab<br>125, 250 mg/5 ml susp | PO | 15 mg/kg/day<br>(otitis 30) | q12h |
| Ceftazidime<br>Ceptaz®, Fortaz®,<br>Tazicef®, Tazidime® | 0.5-, 1-, 2-g vial | IV, IM | 100–150 mg/kg/day<br>(meningitis 150; serious *Pseudo-monas* infection? 200–300) | q8h |
| Ceftibuten<br>Cedax® | 400-mg cap<br>90, 180 mg/5 ml susp | PO | 9 mg/kg/day | q24h |
| Ceftizoxime sodium<br>Cefizox® | 1-, 2-g vial | IV, IM | 150–200 mg/kg/day | q6–8h |
| Ceftriaxone sodium<br>Rocephin® | 0.25-, 0.5-, 1-, 2-g vial | IM, IV | 50–75 mg/kg/day<br>(meningitis 100) | q12–24h |
| Cefuroxime axetil<br>Ceftin® | 125-, 250-, 500-mg tab<br>125, 250 mg/5 ml susp | PO | 20 mg/kg/day (30 for otitis, impetigo) | q12h |
| Cefuroxime sodium<br>Kefurox®, Zinacef® | 0.75-, 1.5-g vial | IV, IM | 100–150 mg/kg/day<br>(meningitis 240) | q8h<br>q6h |
| Cephalexin<br>Keflex®, Keftab®, generic | 250-, 500-mg tab<br>0.25-, 0.5-, 1-g cap<br>100 mg/ml drops<br>125, 250 mg/5 ml susp | PO | 25–50 mg/kg/day | q6–8h |
| Cephalothin sodium<br>Keflin®, Seffin® | 1-, 2-, 4-g vial | IM, IV | 75–125 mg/kg/day | q4–6h |

| | | | | |
|---|---|---|---|---|
| Cephradine<br>Cefadyl®, generic | 0.25-, 0.5-, 1-g vial | IM, IV | 50–100 mg/kg/day | q6h |
| Chloramphenicol sodium succinate<br>Chloromycetin®, generic | 1-g vial | IV | 50–75 mg/kg/day<br>(meningitis 75–100) | q6h |
| Chloroquine HCl<br>Aralen HCl® | 250-mg amp (equiv to 200 mg base) | IM | 5 mg base/kg | 1 or 2 doses |
| Chloroquine $PO_4$<br>Aralen $PO_4$®, generic | 500-mg tab (equiv to 300 mg base) | PO | 10 mg base/kg/day | q24h |
| Chloroquine, hydroxy<br>Plaquenil® | 200-mg tab (equiv to 155 mg base) | PO | 10 mg base/kg/day | q24h |
| Cinoxacin | 250-, 500-mg cap | PO | 1 g/day (adult dose) | q6–12h |
| Ciprofloxacin<br>Cipro® | 100-, 250-, 500-, 750-mg tab<br>50, 100 mg/ml susp | PO | (?) 30–40 mg/kg/day<br>(Not approved for patients < 18 yrs, except for cystic fibrosis) | q12h |
| | 200-, 400-mg vial | IV | | |
| Clarithromycin<br>Biaxin® | 250-, 500-mg tab<br>125, 250 mg/5 ml susp | PO | 15 mg/kg/day | q12h |
| Clindamycin HCl | 75-, 150-, 300-mg cap | PO | 10–20 mg/kg/day | q6–8h |
| Clindamycin palmitate HCl | 75 mg/5 ml solution | PO | 10–20 mg/kg/day | q6–8h |

| Generic and Trade Names | Dosage Form | Route | Dosage | Interval |
|---|---|---|---|---|
| Clindamycin phosphate<br>Cleocin®, generic | 0.3-, 0.6-, 0.9-g vial | IM, IV | 20–40 mg/kg/day | q6–8h |
| Clofazimine<br>Lamprene® | 50-mg cap | PO | 100 mg/day<br>(adult dosage) | q24h |
| Clotrimazole<br>Mycelex® troche | 10-mg lozenge | PO | 10 mg, dissolve in mouth 5 times daily | — |
| Cloxacillin, sodium<br>Cloxapen®, generic | 250-, 500-mg cap<br>125 mg/5 ml solution | PO | 50–100 mg/kg/day | q6h |
| Colistimethate, sodium<br>Coly-Mycin M® | 150-mg vial | IM, IV | 5–7 mg/kg/day | q8h |
| Colistin sulfate<br>Coly-Micin S® | 25 mg/5 ml susp | PO | 15 mg/kg/day | q8h |
| Cycloserine<br>Seromycin® | 250-mg cap | PO | (?) 7–10 mg/kg/day (no established dosage for children) | q12h |
| Dapsone | 25-, 100-mg scored tab | PO | 1 mg/kg/day | q24h |
| Delavirdine<br>Rescriptor® | 100-mg tab | PO | 400 mg t.i.d. (adult dosage) | q8h |
| Demeclocycline HCl<br>Declomycin® | 150-, 300-mg tab | PO | 8–12 mg/kg/day<br>(patients > 7 yrs) | q6–12h |
| Dicloxacillin sodium<br>Dynapen®, generic | 125-, 250-, 500-mg cap<br>62.5 mg/5 ml susp | PO | 12–25 mg/kg/day | q6h |

| | | | | |
|---|---|---|---|---|
| Didanosine (ddI) Videx® | 25-, 50-, 100-, 150-mg chewable tab<br>100-, 167-, 250-, 375-mg, and 2-, 4-g powder for oral solution | PO | 180 mg/m²/day | q12h |
| Diiodohydroxyquin (See Iodoquinol) | | | | |
| Dirithromycin Dynabac® | 250-mg tab | PO | 500 mg (adults; not approved for children) | q24h |
| Doxycycline Doryx®, Vibramycin®, Vibra-Tabs®, generic | 50-, 100-mg cap<br>100-mg tab<br>25 mg/5 ml susp<br>50 mg/5 ml syrup | PO | 2–4 mg/kg/day (patients > 7 yrs) | q12h on 1st day; then ½ dose q24h |
| | 100-mg vial | IV | 2–4 mg/kg/day (patients > 7 yrs) | q24h as 2-hr infusion |
| Enoxacin Penetrex® | 200-, 400-mg tab | PO | 400–800 mg/day (adult dosage) | q12h |
| Erythromycin ERYC®, generic | 250-mg cap, delayed release | PO | 40 mg/kg/day | q6h |
| PCE Dispertab® | 333-, 500-mg tab, delayed release | | | |
| E-Mycin®, Ery-Tab® | 250-, 333-, 500-mg tab, delayed release, enteric coated | | | |
| Erythromycin Base Filmtab® | 250-, 500-mg tab, film coated | | | |

| Generic and Trade Names | Dosage Form | Route | Dosage | Interval |
|---|---|---|---|---|
| Erythromycin estolate<br>Ilosone®, generic | 100 mg/ml drops<br>500-mg tab<br>125-, 250-mg cap<br>125-, 250-mg chewable tab<br>125, 250 mg/5 ml susp | PO | 30–40 mg/kg/day | q8–12h |
| Erythromycin ethylsuccinate<br>E.E.S.®, EryPed®, generic | 400-mg tab<br>200-mg chewable tab<br>200, 400 mg/5 ml susp<br>100 mg/2.5 ml drops | PO | 40 mg/kg/day | q8h |
| Erythromycin ethylsuccinate and sulfisoxazole acetyl<br>Pediazole®, Eryzole®, generic | 200 mg erythromycin and 600 mg sulfisoxazole/5 ml susp | PO | 40 mg/kg/day of erythromycin component | q6–8h |
| Erythromycin lactobionate | 0.5-, 1-g vial | IV | 20–40 mg/kg/day | q6h<br>(1- to 2-hr infusion) |
| Erythromycin stearate<br>Erythrocin®, generic | 250-, 500-mg tab | PO | 20–40 mg/kg/day | q6–8h |
| Ethambutol hydrochloride<br>Myambutol® | 100-, 400-mg tab | PO | 15 mg/kg/day | q24h |
| Ethionamide<br>Trecator-SC® | 250-mg tab | PO | (?) 10–20 mg/kg/day<br>(no established dosage for children) | q12h |

| | | | | |
|---|---|---|---|---|
| Famciclovir<br>Famvir® | 125-, 250-, 500-mg tab | PO | 250 mg for herpes<br>1,500 mg for zoster<br>(adult dosages) | q12h<br>q8h |
| Fansidar<br>(See Sulfadoxine and Pyrimethamine) | | | | |
| Fluconazole<br>Diflucan® | 50-, 100-, 200-mg tab<br>50, 200 mg/5 ml susp | PO | 3–6 mg/kg/day<br>(max 600 mg/day) | q24h |
| | 200-, 400-mg vial | IV | | |
| Flucytosine<br>Ancobon® | 250-, 500-mg cap | PO | 50–150 mg/kg/day | q6h |
| Foscarnet sodium<br>Foscavir® | 6-, 12-g vial | IV | Initial: 180 mg/kg/day<br>Maintenance: 90–120 mg/kg/day | q8h<br>q24h |
| Furazolidone<br>Furoxone® | 100-mg tab<br>50 mg/15 ml (17 mg/5 ml) susp | PO | 5–8 mg/kg/day | q6h |
| Ganciclovir sodium<br>Cytovene® | 500-mg vial<br>250-mg cap | IV<br>PO | Induction: 10 mg/kg/day<br>(1–2 hrs IV infusion)<br>Maintenance: 5 mg/kg/day (no established dosage for children) | q12h<br>q24h |
| Gentamicin sulfate<br>Garamycin®, generic | 20-, 80-mg vial | IM, IV | 3–7.5 mg/kg/day (cystic fibrosis 7–10); (See page 4 regarding q24h dosing) | q8h |
| Grepafloxacin<br>Raxar® | 200-mg tab | PO | 400–600 mg/day (adults; not approved for patients < 18 yrs) | q24h |

| Generic and Trade Names | Dosage Form | Route | Dosage | Interval |
| --- | --- | --- | --- | --- |
| Griseofulvin<br>Fulvicin-P/G®, Grifulvin V®, Grisactin®, Gris-PEG® | Microsize: 250-, 500-mg tab<br>125 mg/5 ml susp | PO | 15 mg/kg/day | q24h |
| | Ultramicrosize: 125-, 165-, 250-, 330-mg tab | | 6–7 mg/kg/day | q12–24h |
| Imipenem-Cilastatin sodium<br>Primaxin® | 250/250-, 500/500-mg vial (IV)<br>500/500-, 750/750-mg vial (IM) | IM, IV | 60–100 mg/kg/day | q6h |
| Indinavir<br>Crixivan® | 200-, 400-mg cap | PO | 800 mg t.i.d. (adult dosage) | q8h |
| Iodoquinol<br>Yodoxin® | 210-, 650-mg tab | PO | 40 mg/kg/day | q8h |
| Isoniazid<br>Nydrazid®, generic | 150-, 300-mg cap<br>100-, 300-mg scored tab<br>1-g vial | PO, IM | 50 mg/5 ml syrup<br>10–20 mg/kg/day (max 300 mg) | q12–24h |
| Itraconazole<br>Sporanox® | 100-mg cap<br>10 mg/ml solution | PO | 200–400 mg/day (adult dosage)<br>? 5 mg/kg/day | q24h |
| Ivermectin<br>Stromectal® | 6-mg scored tab | PO | 150–200 mcg/kg | 1 dose |
| Kanamycin sulfate<br>Kantrex®, generic | 75-mg, 0.5-, 1-g vial | IM, IV | 15–30 mg/kg/day (see page 4 regarding q24h dosing) | q8h |
| | 500-mg cap | PO | 150–250 mg/kg/day (for suppression of bowel flora) | q1–6h |

| | | | | |
|---|---|---|---|---|
| Ketoconazole<br>Nizoral® | 200-mg scored tab | PO | 3.3–6.6 mg/kg/day (max 800 mg/day) | q24h |
| Lamivudine<br>Epivir® | 150-mg tab<br>50 mg/5 ml solution | PO | 8 mg/kg/day | q12h |
| Levofloxacin<br>Levaquin® | 250-, 500-mg tab<br>500-mg vial | PO<br>IV | 500 mg/day (adults; not approved for patients < 18 yrs) | q24h |
| Lomefloxacin HCl<br>Maxaquin® | 400-mg scored tab | PO | 400 mg/day (adults; not approved for patients < 18 yrs) | q24h |
| Loracarbef<br>Lorabid® | 200-, 400-mg cap<br>100, 200 mg/5 ml susp | PO | 30 (otitis)–15 (other indications) mg/kg/day | q12h |
| Mebendazole<br>Vermox® | 100-mg chewable tab | PO | See Section VII | |
| Mefloquine HCl<br>Lariam® | 250-mg scored tab | PO | See Section VII | |
| Meropenem<br>Merrem® | 0.5-, 1-g vial | IV | 60 mg/kg/day<br>(meningitis 120) | q8h |
| Methenamine hippurate<br>Urex® | 1-g tab | PO | 25–50 mg/kg/day | q12h |
| Methenamine mandelate<br>Uroquid®, generic | 500-mg tab<br>500 mg/5 ml susp | PO | 50–75 mg/kg/day | q6h |
| Metronidazole<br>Flagyl®, generic | 250-, 500-mg tab | PO | 15–35 mg/kg/day | q8h |
| | 500-mg vial | IV | 30 mg/kg/day | q6h |

| Generic and Trade Names | Dosage Form | Route | Dosage | Interval |
|---|---|---|---|---|
| Mezlocillin sodium Mezlin® | 1-, 2-, 3-, 4-g vial | IV | 200–300 mg/kg/day | q4–6h |
| Miconazole Monistat® | 200-mg amp | IV | 20–40 mg/kg/day | q8h |
| Minocycline HCl Dynacin®, Minocin®, generic | 50-, 100-mg pellet-filled cap<br>50 mg/5 ml susp | PO | 4 mg/kg/day (patients > 7 yrs) | q12h |
| | 100-mg vial | IV | 4 mg/kg/day (patients > 7 yrs) | q12h |
| Mupirocin Bactroban®, Bactroban Nasal | 15-, 30-g tube<br>1-g tube (nasal) | Topical | Apply to infected skin or nasal mucosa | q8h |
| Nafcillin sodium Unipen® | 250-mg cap, 500-mg tab, 250 mg/5 ml solution | PO | 50–100 mg/kg/day | q6h |
| | 0.5-, 1-, 2-g vial | IM, IV | 150 mg/kg/day | q6h |
| Nalidixic acid NegGram® | 0.25-, 0.5-, 1-g tab<br>250 mg/5 ml susp | PO | 55 mg/kg/day | q6h |
| Nelfinavir Viracept® | 250-mg tab<br>50 mg/g oral powder | PO | 750 mg t.i.d. or 1250 mg b.i.d. (adult dosage) | q8–12h |
| Neomycin sulfate | 500-mg tab<br>125 mg/5 ml solution | PO | 50–100 mg/kg/day | q6–8h |

| | | | | |
|---|---|---|---|---|
| Netilmicin sulfate<br>Netromycin® | 150-mg vial | IV, IM | 3–7.5 mg/kg/day; (See page 4 regarding q24h dosing) | q8h |
| Nevirapine<br>Viramune® | 200-mg tab | PO | 200 mg b.i.d. (adult dosage) | q12h |
| Nitrofurantoin<br>Furadantin® | 25 mg/5 ml susp | PO | 5–7 mg/kg/day | q6h |
| Nitrofurantoin<br>Macrodantin®, generic | 25-, 50-, 100-mg cap | PO | 5–7 mg/kg/day | q6h |
| Norfloxacin<br>Noroxin® | 400-mg tab | PO | 800 mg/day (adults; not approved for patients < 18 yrs) | q12h |
| Nystatin<br>Mycostatin®, generic | 100,000 U/ml susp<br>500,000-U tab | PO (not swallowed) | Infants 2 ml/dose; Children 4–6 ml or 1 tab/dose | q6h |
| Ofloxacin<br>Floxin® | 200-, 300-, 400-mg tab<br>400-mg vial | PO | 400–800 mg/day (adult dosage) | q12h |
| Oxacillin, sodium | 250-, 500-mg cap<br>250 mg/5 ml solution | PO | 50–100 mg/kg/day | q6h |
| | 0.25-, 0.5-, 1-, 2-, 4-g vial | IM, IV | 150–200 mg/kg/day | q6h |
| Oxytetracycline HCl<br>Terramycin® | 500-mg vial with 2% lidocaine | IM | 15–25 mg/kg/day | q8–12h |
| Palivizumab<br>Synagis® | 100-mg vial | IM | 15 mg/kg once monthly (for prophylaxis) | Monthly |
| Paromomycin sulfate<br>Humatin®, generic | 250-mg cap | PO | 30 mg/kg/day | q8h |

| Generic and Trade Names | Dosage Form | Route | Dosage | Interval |
|---|---|---|---|---|
| Penicillin G, benzathine Bicillin® | 3-million-U 10-ml vial; 1-, 1.5-, and 2-ml syringes containing 600,000 U/ml | IM | 50,000 U/kg | 1 dose |
| Penicillin G, potassium Pfizerpen® | 1-, 2-, 10-, 20-million-U vial | IV | 100,000–250,000 U/kg/day | q4h |
| Penicillin G, procaine Wycillin® | 0.3-, 0.6-, 1.2-, 2.4-million-U vial | IM | 25,000–50,000 U/kg/day | q12–24h |
| | 5-million-U vial | IM, IV | 100,000–250,000 U/kg/day | q4h |
| Penicillin V Pen-Vee K®, Veetids®, generic | 125-, 250-, 500-mg tab<br>125, 250 mg/5 ml solution<br>125, 250 mg/5 ml drops | PO | 25–50 mg/kg/day | q6–8h |
| Pentamidine isethionate | 300-mg vial | IV | 4 mg/kg/day | q24h |
| Piperacillin sodium Pipracil® | 2-, 3-, 4-g vial | IV | 200–300 mg/kg/day (not approved for children) | q4–6h |
| Piperacillin/Tazobactam Zosyn® | 2/.25-, 3/.375-, 4/.5-g vial | IV | 240 mg PIP/kg/day (not approved for children) | q4–6h |
| Praziquantel Biltricide® | 600-mg triscored tab | PO | 50–75 mg/kg/day | q8h |
| Pyrazinamide | 500-mg tab | PO | 30 mg/kg/day | q12–24h |
| Pyrimethamine (See Sulfadoxine) Daraprim® | 25-mg scored tab | PO | 0.5–1 mg/kg/day | q12h |

| | | | | |
|---|---|---|---|---|
| Quinacrine HCl (Not available in the United States) | 100-mg cap | PO | 6 mg/kg/day | q8h |
| Ribavirin<br>Virazole® | 6-g vial | nhalation | 1 vial by SPAG-2 aerosol generator | q24h |
| | 200-mg cap for use with interferon-2β also available as Rebetol® | PO | 1000–1200 mg/day (adult dosage) | q12h |
| Rifabutin<br>Mycobutin® | 150-mg cap | PO | 300 mg/day (adult dosage) | q12–24h |
| Rifampin<br>Rifadin®, Rimactane® | 150-, 300-mg cap<br>600-mg vial | PO<br>IV | 10–20 mg/kg/day<br>(max 600 mg) | q12–24h |
| Rifapentine<br>Priftin® | 150-mg tab | PO | 600 mg twice weekly (adult dosage) | — |
| Rimantadine HCl<br>Flumadine® | 100-mg tab<br>50 mg/5 ml syrup | PO | 5 mg/kg/day<br>(max 150 mg/day) | q12–24h |
| Ritonavir<br>Norvir® | 100-mg cap<br>80 mg/ml oral solution | PO | 1200 mg/day (adult dosage) | q12h |
| Saquinavir mesylate<br>Invirase® | 200-mg cap | PO | 1800 mg/day (adult dosage) | q8h |
| Sparfloxacin<br>Zagam® | 200-mg tab | PO | 400 mg 1st dose; then 200 mg/day (adults; not approved for patients < 18 yrs) | q24h |
| Spectinomycin HCl<br>Trobicin® | 2-, 4-g vial | IM | 30–40 mg/kg | 1 dose |

| Generic and Trade Names | Dosage Form | Route | Dosage | Interval |
|---|---|---|---|---|
| Stavudine (d4T)<br>Zerit® | 15-, 20-, 30-, 40-mg cap<br>5 mg/5 ml solution | PO | 2 mg/kg/day | q12h |
| Streptomycin sulfate<br>Microsulfon®, generic | 1-g vial | IM | 20–30 mg/kg/day | q12h |
| Sulfadiazine | 0.3-, 0.5-g tab | PO | 120–150 mg/kg/day | q4–6h |
| Sulfadoxine and pyrimeth-amine<br>Fansidar® | 500-mg SDX + 25-mg PMA scored tab | PO | See Section VII | |
| Sulfamethoxazole<br>Gantanol®, generic | 0.5-g tab<br>0.5 g/5 ml susp | PO | 50–60 mg/kg/day | q12h |
| Sulfasalazine<br>Azulfidine®, generic | 500-mg tab | PO | 30–60 mg/kg/day | q4–8h |
| Sulfisoxazole<br>Gantrisin®, generic | 0.5-g tab<br>0.5 g/5 ml susp or syrup | PO | 120–150 mg/kg/day | q4–6h |
| Terbinafine<br>Lamisil® | 250-mg tab | PO | 250 mg/day (adults; not approved for children) | q24h |
| Tetracycline<br>Achromycin®, Panmycin®, Sumycin®, generic | 250-, 500-mg cap | PO | 25–50 mg/kg/day<br>(patients > 7 yrs) | q6h |
| Thalidomide<br>Thalomid® | 50-mg cap | PO | Restricted to specially licensed prescribers (for leprosy) | q24h |

| | | | | |
|---|---|---|---|---|
| Thiabendazole<br>Mintezol® | 500-mg chewable, scored tab<br>500 mg/5 ml susp | PO | 50 mg/kg/day | q12h |
| Ticarcillin disodium<br>Ticar® | 1-, 3-, 6-g vial | IV | 200–300 mg/kg/day | q4–6h |
| Ticarcillin and clavulanate potassium<br>Timentin® | 3/0.1-, 3/0.2-g vial | IV | 200–300 mg/kg/day | q4–6h |
| Tobramycin sulfate<br>Nebcin®, generic | 20-, 80-mg, 1.2-g vial | IV, IM | 3–7.5 mg/kg/day (cystic fibrosis 7–10); (See page 4 regarding q24h dosing) | q8h |
| Trifluridine<br>Viroptic® | 1% ophthalmic solution | Topical | 1 drop (max 9 drops/day) | q2h |
| Trimethoprim<br>Trimpex®, generic | 100-mg scored tab | PO | 4–10 mg/kg/day (not approved for children) | q12h |
| Trimethoprim-Sulfa-methoxazole<br>Bactrim®, Septra®, generic | 80-mg TMP/400-mg SMX tab<br>160-mg TMP/800-mg SMX tab<br>40-mg TMP/200-mg SMX/5 ml susp | PO | 8–12-mg TMP/40–60-mg SMX/kg/day; (20-mg TMP/100-mg SMX/kg/day for *Pneumocystis*) | q12h |
| | 400-mg TMP/2000-mg SMX amp | IV | | q6h |
| Trimetrexate glucuronate<br>Neutrexin® | 25 mg/5 ml vial | IV | 45 mg/m$^2$ (adult dose); Must be given with leucovorin | q24h |
| Troleandomycin<br>Tao® | 250-mg cap | PO | 25–40 mg/kg/day | q6h |

| Generic and Trade Names | Dosage Form | Route | Dosage | Interval |
|---|---|---|---|---|
| Valacyclovir HCl<br>Valtrex® | 500-mg, 1-g cap | PO | Herpes simplex: 1000 mg/day<br>Herpes zoster: 3000 mg/day (adult dosage) | q12h |
| Vancomycin HCl<br>Vancocin®, generic | 1-, 10-g bottle<br>125-, 250-mg cap | PO | 40 mg/kg/day (oral use not recommended) | q6–8h |
| | 0.5-, 1-g vial | IV | 40 mg/kg/day (meningitis 60) as 1 hr infusion | q6h |
| Vidarabine<br>Vira-A® | 3% ophthalmic ointment | Topical | Approximately 1 cm of ointment | q3h |
| Zalcitabine (ddC)<br>HIVID® | 0.375-, 0.750-mg tab | PO | 2.25 mg/day (adult dosage) | q8h |
| Zidovudine (AZT)<br>Retrovir® | 200-mg vial<br>100-mg cap<br>50 mg/5 ml syrup | IV<br>PO | 480 mg/m$^2$/day (max 600 mg/day) | q6h |

# IX. ALPHABETICAL LISTING OF TRADE NAMES

**Trade Name** (Drug Company)
—Generic Name

-A-

**ABELCET** (Liposome Company)
—amphotericin B, lipid complex
**Achromycin** (Lederle)
—tetracycline
**Agenerase** (Glaxo Wellcome)
—amprenavir
**Albenza** (SmithKline Beecham)
—albendazole
**AmBisome** (Fujisawa)
—amphotericin B liposome
**Amoxil** (SmithKline Beecham)
—amoxicillin
**AMPHOTEC** (Sequus)
—amphotericin B cholesteryl sulfate
**Ancef** (SmithKline Beecham)
—cefazolin
**Ancobon** (ICN)
—flucytosine
**Aralen** (Sanofi)
—cloroquine
**Aralen with Primaquine** (Sanofi)
—cloroquine/primaquine
**A/T/S** (Hoechst Marion Roussel)
—2% erythromycin solution (topical)
**Augmentin** (SmithKline Beecham)
—amoxicillin/clavulanate potassium
**Azactam** (Bristol-Myers Squibb)
—aztreonam
**Azulfidine** (Pharmacia & Upjohn)
—sulfasalazine

-B-

**Bactrim** (Roche)
—trimethoprim/sulfamethoxazole
**Bactroban** (SmithKline Beecham)
—mupirocin (topical)
**Benemid** (Merck)
—probenecid
**Biaxin** (Abbott)
—clarithromycin
**Bicillin** (Wyeth-Ayerst)
—benzathine penicillin G
**Biltricide** (Bayer)
—praziquantel

-C-

**Ceclor** (Lilly)
—cefaclor
**Cedax** (Schering)
—ceftibuten
**Cefadyl** (Apothecon)
—cephradine
**Cefizox** (Fujisawa)
—ceftizoxime
**Cefobid** (Pfizer)
—cefoperazone
**Cefotan** (Astra Zeneca)
—cefotetan
**Ceftin** (Glaxo Wellcome)
—cefuroxime axetil
**Cefzil** (Bristol-Myers Squibb)
—cefprozil
**Ceptaz** (Glaxo Wellcome)
—ceftazidime
**Chibroxin** (Merck)
—norfloxacin ophthalmic solution
**Chloromycetin** (Parke-Davis)
—chloramphenicol
**Cinobac** (Oclassen)
—cinoxacin
**Cipro** (Bayer)
—ciprofloxacin
**Claforan** (Hoechst Marion Roussel)
—cefotaxime
**Cleocin** (Pharmacia & Upjohn)
—clindamycin
**Cloxapen** (SmithKline Beecham)
—cloxacillin
**Coly-Mycin** (Monarch)
—colistin
**Combivir** (Glaxo Wellcome)
—zidovudine + lamivudine
**Cytovene** (Roche)
—ganciclovir

-D-

**Dapsone USP** (Jacobus)
—dapsone
**Daraprim** (Glaxo Wellcome)
—pyrimethamine

**Declomycin** (Lederle)
—demeclocycline
**Denavir** (SmithKline Beecham)
—penciclovir 1% cream
**Diflucan** (Pfizer)
—fluconazole
**Doryx** (Warner Chilcott)
—doxycycline
**Duricef** (Bristol-Myers Squibb)
—cefadroxil
**Dynabac** (Sanofi)
—dirithromycin
**DYNACIN** (Medicis)
—minocycline
**Dynapen** (Apothecon)
—dicloxacillin

-E-

**E. E. S.** (Abbott)
—erythromycin ethylsuccinate
**Elimite Cream** (Allergan)
—permethrin 5% (topical)
**E-Mycin** (Knoll)
—Erythromycin
**Epivir** (Glaxo Wellcome)
—lamivudine
**ERYC** (Warner Chilcott)
—erythromycin
**Erygel** (Allergan)
—2% erythromycin gel (topical)
**EryPed** (Abbott)
—erythromycin ethylsuccinate
**Ery-Tab** (Abbott)
—erythromycin
**Erythrocin** (Abbott)
—erythromycin stearate
**Eryzole** (Alra)
—erythromycin ethylsuccinate/sulfisoxazole acetyl

-F-

**Famvir** (SmithKline Beecham)
—famciclovir
**Fansidar** (Roche)
—sulfadoxine/pyrimethamine
**Flagyl** (Searle)
—metronidazole
**Floxin** (Ortho-McNeil)
—ofloxacin
**Flumadine** (Forest)
—rimantadine
**Fortaz** (Glaxo Wellcome)
—ceftazidime
**Fortovase** (Roche)
—saquinavir
**Foscavir** (Astra)
—foscarnet
**Fulvicin** (Schering)
—griseofulvin
**Fungizone** (Bristol-Myers Squibb)
—amphotericin B
**Furadantin** (Dura)
—nitrofurantoin
**Furoxone** (Roberts)
—furazolidone

-G-

**Gantanol** (Roche)
—sulfamethoxazole
**Gantrisin** (Roche)
—sulfisoxazole
**Garamycin** (Schering)
—gentamicin
**Geocillin** (Pfizer)
—carbenicillin indanyl
**Grifulvin V** (Ortho)
—griseofulvin
**Grisactin** (Wyeth-Ayerst)
—griseofulvin
**Gris-PEG** (Allergan)
—griseofulvin

-H-

**HIVID** (Roche)
—zalcitabine
**Humatin** (Monarch)
—paromomycin

-I-

**Ilosone** (Dista)
—erythromycin estolate
**Ilotycin** (Dista)
—erythromycin
**Invirase** (Roche)
—saquinavir

-K-

**Kantrex** (Apothecon)
—kanamycin
**Keflex** (Dista)
—cephalexin

**Keflin** (Lilly)
—cephalothin
**Keftab** (Dura)
—cephalexin
**Kefurox** (Lilly)
—cefuroxime
**Kefzol** (Lilly)
—cefazolin

-L-

**Lamprene** (Novartis)
—clofazimine
**Lariam** (Roche)
—mefloquine
**Levaquin** (Ortho-McNeil)
—levofloxacin
**Lincocin** (Pharmacia & Upjohn)
—lincomycin
**Lorabid** (Lilly)
—loracarbef
**Lotrimin** (Schering)
—clotrimazole (topical)

-M-

**Macrodantin** (Procter & Gamble)
—nitrofurantoin
**Mandol** (Lilly)
—cefamandole
**Maxaquin** (Unimed)
—lomefloxacin
**Maxipime** (Bristol-Myers Squibb)
—cefipime
**Mefoxin** (Merck)
—cefoxitin
**Mepron** (Glaxo Wellcome)
—atovaquone
**Merrem** (Astra Zeneca)
—meropenem
**Mezlin** (Bayer)
—mezlocillin
**Microsulfor** (Eli Lilly)
—sulfadiazine
**Minocin** (Lederle)
—minocycline
**Mintezol** (Merck)
—thiabendazole
**Monistat** (Ortho)
—miconazole
**Monocid** (SmithKline Beecham)
—cefonicid
**Monural** (Forest)
—fosfomycin tromethamine
**Myambutol** (Lederle)
—ethambutol
**Mycelex** (Bayer; Alza)
—clotrimazole
**Mycobutin** (Pharmacia & Upjohn)
—rifabutin
**Mycostatin** (Bristol-Myers Squibb)
—nystatin

-N-

**Nebcin** (Lilly)
—tobramycin
**NegGram** (Sanofi)
—nalidixic acid
**Neosporin** (Warner Lambert)
—neomycin, polymyxin B (topical)
**Netromycin** (Schering)
—netilmicin
**Neutrexin** (U.S. Bioscience)
—trimetrexate
**Nix Creme Rinse** (Warner Lambert)
—permethrim 1% (topical)
**Nizoral** (Janssen)
—ketoconazole
**Noroxin** (Merck; Roberts)
—norfloxacin
**Norvir** (Abbott)
—ritonavir
**Nydrazid** (Apothecon)
—isoniazid

-O-

**Omnicef** (Parke Davis)
—cefdinir
**Omnipen** (Wyeth-Ayerst)
—ampicillin

-P-

**Panmycin** (Pharmacia & Upjohn)
—tetracycline
**PCE Dispertab** (Abbott)
—erythromycin particles in tablets
**Pediazole** (Ross)
—erythromycin ethylsuccinate/ sulfisoxazole acetyl
**Penetrex** (Rhone-Poulenc Rorer)
—enoxacin
**Pen-Vee K** (Wyeth-Ayerst)
—penicillin V
**Pfizerpen** (Pfizer)
—penicillin G

**Pipracil** (Lederle)
—piperacillin
**Plaquenil** (Sanofi)
—hydroxychloroquine
**Polysporin** (Warner Lambert)
—polymyxin B/bacitracin (topical)
**Polytrim Ophthalmic Solution** (Allergan)
—trimethoprim and polymyxin B (topical)
**Preveon** (Gilead)
—adefovir
**Priftin** (Hoechst Marion Roussel)
—rifapentine
**Primaxin** (Merck)
—imipenem-cilastatin
**Principen** (Apothecon)
—ampicillin
**Pyrazinamide** (Wyeth-Lederle)
—pyrazinamide

-R-

**Raxar** (Glaxo Wellcome)
—grepafloxacin
**Rebetron** (Schering)
—ribavirin and interferon-2b
**Rescriptor** (Pharmacia & Upjohn)
—delavirdine
**Retrovir** (Glaxo Wellcome)
—zidovudine
**Rifadin** (Hoechst Marion Roussel)
—rifampin
**Rifamate** (Hoechst Marion Roussel)
—rifampin/isoniazid
**Rifater** (Hoechst Marion Roussel)
—rifampin, isoniazid, pyrazinamide
**Rimactane** (Geneva)
—rifampin
**Rocephin** (Roche)
—ceftriaxone

-S-

**Seffin** (Glaxo Wellcome)
—cephalothin
**Septra** (Monarch)
—trimethoprim/sulfamethoxazole
**Seromycin** (Dura)
—cycloserine
**Spectrobid** (Pfizer)
—bacampicillin
**Sporanox** (Janssen)
—itraconazole
**Stromectal** (Merck)
—ivermectin
**Sumycin** (Apothecon)
—tetracycline
**Suprax** (Lederle)
—cefixime
**Sustiva** (Dupont)
—efavirenz
**Symmetrel** (Endo)
—amantadine
**Synagis** (MedImmune)
—palivizumab

-T-

**Tao** (Pfizer)
—troleandomycin
**Tazicef** (SmithKline Beecham)
—ceftazidime
**Tazidime** (Lilly)
—ceftazidime
**Terramycin** (Pfizer)
—oxytetracycline
**Thalomid** (Celgene)
—thalidomide
**Tlcar** (SmithKline Beecham)
—ticarcillin
**Tice BCG Vaccine** (Organon)
—BCG Vaccine
**Timentin** (SmithKline Beecham)
—ticarcillin/clavulanate
**Trecator-SC** (Wyeth-Ayerst)
—ethionamide
**Trimox** (Apothecon)
—amoxicillin
**Trimpex** (Roche)
—trimethoprim
**Trobicin** (Pharmacia & Upjohn)
—spectinomycin
**Trovan** (Pfizer)
—trovafloxacin

-U-

**Unasyn** (Pfizer)
—ampicillin/sulbactam
**Urex** (3M)
—methenamine hipprate
**Urobiotic** (Pfizer)
—oxytetracycline, sulfamethizole/phenazopyridine
**Uroquid-Acid** (Beach)
—methenamine/sodium acid phosphate

-V-

**Valtrex** (Glaxo Wellcome)
—valacyclovir
**Vancocin** (Lilly)
—vancomycin
**Vantin** (Pharmacia & Upjohn)
—cefpodoxime proxetil
**Veetids** (Apothecon)
—penicillin V
**Vermox** (Janssen)
—mebendazole
**Vibramycin** (Pfizer)
—doxycycline
**Vibra-Tabs** (Pfizer)
—doxycycline
**Videx** (Bristol-Myers Squibb)
—didanosine
**Vira-A** (Monarch)
—vidarabine
**Viracept** (Agouron)
—nelfinavir
**Viramune** (Roxane)
—nevirapine
**Virazole** (ICN)
—ribavirin
**Viroptic** (Glaxo Wellcome)
—trifluridine (Ophthalmic)

-W-

**Wycillin** (Wyeth-Ayerst)
—penicillin G procaine
**Wymox** (Wyeth-Ayerst)
—amoxicillin

-Y-

**Yodoxin** (Glenwood)
—iodoquinol (formerly diiodohydroxyquin)

-Z-

**Zagam** (Rhône-Poulenc Rorer)
—sparfloxacin
**Zerit** (Bristol-Myers Squibb)
—stavudine
**Ziagen** (Glaxo Wellcome)
—abacavir
**Zinacef** (Glaxo Wellcome)
—cefuroxime
**Zithromax** (Pfizer)
—azithromycin
**Zosyn** (Lederle)
—piperacillin/tazobactam
**Zovirax** (Glaxo Wellcome)
—acyclovir

## X. PENICILLIN DESENSITIZATION

Because of the numerous alternative available antibiotics, desensitization to penicillin or other beta-lactam drugs is rarely needed. Studies have shown that an oral regimen is safer and more effective for desensitization to penicillins than graduated injections (Pediatr Infect Dis 1982;1:344).

Penicillin V suspension is used. Signed, informed consent is required. An intravenous catheter is in place and emergency resuscitation materials at hand for the unlikely event of anaphylaxis. Medical personnel capable of managing anaphylaxis should be available. Doses are given at 15-minute intervals; the total regimen requires 4 hours.

| | Penicillin V | |
|---|---|---|
| Doses | mg/ml | Amount q15min |
| 1–7 | 0.5 | Doubling doses from 0.1 ml (0.05 mg) to 6.4 ml (3.2 mg) units |
| 8–10 | 10,000 | Doubling doses from 1.2 ml (6 mg) to 4.8 ml (24 mg) |
| 11–14 | 80,000 | Doubling doses from 1.0 ml (50 mg) to 8.0 ml (400 mg) |

(Sources: N Engl J Med 1985;312:1229; Middleton E, et al. [eds]. Allergy: Principles and Practice, 4th ed. Baltimore: Mosby, 1993, p. 1738.)

Minor allergic reactions are suppressed with epinephrine or antihistamines. Therapy is not interrupted unless there is a severe or unsuppressible reaction. If there are interruptions in therapy of more than 8 hours, it is advisable to repeat the desensitization regimen.

For other beta-lactam antibiotics, the same regimen can be used as that outlined above for penicillin.

## XI. SEQUENTIAL PARENTERAL-ORAL ANTIBIOTIC THERAPY FOR SERIOUS INFECTIONS

Bacterial pneumonias, bone and joint infections, and deep tissue abscesses often require prolonged antibiotic therapy. Intravenous therapy is unpleasant for the child and carries a hazard of nosocomial infection during hospitalization.

**Rationale:**

1. Comparable dosages of analogous parenteral and oral medications result in comparable serum concentrations 1–6 hours after a dose and comparable bioavailability ("area-under-the-curve") in most patients.
2. No known therapeutic advantage exists to the momentary high serum concentrations that occur during IV administration.
3. The majority of organisms are removed by the initial parenteral therapy and by surgical drainage. Large dosage oral therapy eradicates remaining pathogens when tissue perfusion is improved.

**Method:**

1. Initial parenteral therapy is as follows:
   a. Alert laboratory to save pathogen for serum bactericidal tests.
   b. Perform any necessary surgical procedures.
2. Subsequent oral therapy when clinical condition is stable and patient can take and retain oral medication (usually 5–7 days) is as follows:
   a. Select appropriate oral antibiotic based on *in vitro* susceptibilities and compliance factors (mainly palatability of suspension formulations).
   b. BEGIN WITH DOSAGE TWO TO THREE TIMES "NORMAL" DOSAGE (e.g., 75–100 mg/kg/day OF DICLOXACILLIN AND 100–150 mg/kg/day OF OTHER BETA-LACTAMS).
   c. Serum for bactericidal titer or measurement of antibiotic concentration 1–2 hours after a dose.

**NOTES:**

1. The serum bactericidal titer is done quantitatively and is defined as $\geq$ 99.9% killing. For staphylococcal infections the serum bactericidal titer should be at least 1:8. Peak serum antibiotic concentration should be $\geq$ 20 g/ml for beta-lactams and $\geq$ 10 g/ml for clindamycin. (NOTE: Measuring bactericidal titers is labor-intensive and difficult to standardize. Measuring antibiotic may be preferable.)
2. Peak serum activity usually is found 45–60 minutes after a dose taken as suspension and 1–2 hours after a capsule or tablet.
3. Approximately 5–10% of patients are unsuitable for this regimen because of poor gastrointestinal absorption of antibiotics or poor compliance with taking prescribed medicine. Parenteral therapy is resumed.

**WARNING:** ORAL THERAPY REGIMENS FOR SERIOUS INFECTIONS ARE POTENTIALLY HAZARDOUS UNLESS ADEQUACY OF SERUM BACTERICIDAL ACTIVITY OR ANTIBIOTIC CONTENT IS MONITORED.

# XII. ANTIBIOTIC THERAPY IN PATIENTS WITH RENAL FAILURE

Most antimicrobials are excreted primarily by the kidneys; therefore, when significant renal functional impairment is present, either downward adjustments in dosages must be made or the intervals between doses must be lengthened. Exceptions are drugs such as chloramphenicol that are metabolized to antibiotically inactive conjugates and those excreted primarily by the liver, such as nafcillin and ceftriaxone.

Degrees of dosage adjustment necessary for treating patients with renal failure are as follows: Major adjustments in dosage and dosing intervals are necessary for treating renal failure patients with aminoglycosides, flucytosine, and vancomycin. No adjustments in dosage are necessary in the use of amphotericin B, cefoperazone, chloramphenicol, cloxacillin, dicloxacillin, doxycycline, erythromycin, isoniazid, metronidazole, minocycline, nafcillin, and rifampin. For other antibiotics, minor to moderate adjustments are necessary.

The most satisfactory way to use drugs in children with decreased renal function is by monitoring the antibiotic concentrations in serum. The customary initial loading dose is given. Initially, until antibiotic assay results are available, one makes estimates of appropriate dosage based on past experience of rates of excretion related to the degree of renal failure. Three or four serum specimens are collected at intervals over a 12–24 hour period for assay of antibiotic content. The serum half-life is estimated. The interval of dosing is every three half-lives for patients with moderate renal dysfunction and every two half-lives for those with severe renal failure; subsequent dosages are two-thirds or one-half, respectively, of the initial loading dose.

**CLINICAL PHARMACISTS HAVE COMPUTER PROGRAMS FOR CALCULATING ANTIBIOTIC DOSAGE MODIFICATION BASED ON CREATININE CLEARANCE OR SERUM CREATININE AND CALCULATED SERUM HALF-LIFE.**

Patients undergoing dialysis need additional doses after the procedure if a substantial amount of drug is removed by dialysis. With peritoneal dialysis, less than 10% of the drug is removed in the case of most antibiotics. The exceptions are aminoglycosides (20–25%), cefazolin and cefuroxime (20%), and vancomycin (15–20%).

| Removed by Hemodialysis | Beta-Lactams | Other Drugs |
|---|---|---|
| > 50% | Many cephalosporins (see exceptions below), imipenem | Acyclovir, aminoglycosides, flucytosine, isoniazid, spectinomycin sulfonamides, trimethoprim, fluconazole |
| 20–50% | Most penicillins (see exceptions below), aztreonam, cefaclor, ceforanide, cephapirin | Ethambutol, metronidazole, vancomycin |
| < 10% | Cefixime, cefonicid, cefoperazone, cefotetan, cloxacillin, dicloxacillin, methicillin, nafcillin, oxacillin | Amphotericin B, fluoroquinolones, macrolides, miconazole, polymyxins, tetracyclines |

# XIII. DILUTIONS OF ANTIBIOTICS FOR INTRAVENOUS USE

Sometimes manufacturers' recommendations for dilution of antibiotics for IV use are not appropriate for pediatric patients. These recommendations were prepared by the clinical pharmacists at Children's Medical Center, Dallas.

| | Concentration in mg/ml for: | | |
|---|---|---|---|
| Drug | Central Catheter | Peripheral Vein | Duration of Infusion |
| Acyclovir | 10 | 7 | 1–3 hrs |
| Amikacin | 5 | 5 | 30 mins |
| Amphotericin B | 0.25 | 0.1 | 2–4 hrs |
| Ampicillin | 100 | 50 | ≤ 10 mg/kg/min |
| Azithromycin | 1–2 | 1–2 | 1–2 hrs |
| Aztreonam | 66 | 20 | ≤ 6 mg/kg/min |
| Cefazolin | 125 | 40 | ≤ 6 mg/kg/min |
| Cefepime | 40 | 40 | 30 mins |
| Cefotaxime | 200 | 60 | ≤ 10 mg/kg/min |
| Cefoxitin | 180 | 50 | ≤ 8 mg/kg/min |
| Ceftazidime | 200 | 40 | ≤ 10 mg/kg/min |
| Ceftriaxone | 100 | 50 | ≤ 10 mg/kg/min |
| Cefuroxime | 100 | 50 | ≤ 10 mg/kg/min |
| Chloramphenicol | 100 | 50 | 30 mins |
| Ciprofloxacin | 2 | 2 | 60 mins |
| Clindamycin | 18 | 18 | 15–30 mins |
| Doxycycline | 1 | 1 | 60 mins |
| Erythromycin | 10 | 5 | 60 mins |
| Fluconazole | 2 | 2 | ≤ 3 mg/min |
| Foscarnet | 24 | 12 | 60 mins |
| Ganciclovir | 10 | 10 | 60 mins |

| Drug | Concentration in mg/ml for: Central Catheter | Peripheral Vein | Duration of Infusion |
|---|---|---|---|
| Gentamicin | 40 | 40 | 30 mins |
| Imipenem/cilastatin | 5 | 5 | 30–60 mins |
| Kanamycin | 6 | 5 | 30 mins |
| Meropenem | 50 | 50 | 15–30 mins |
| Metronidazole | 5 | 5 | 60 mins |
| Mezlocillin | 100 | 50 | ≤ 10 mg/kg/min |
| Miconazole | 6 | 6 | 30–60 mins |
| Nafcillin | 100 | 40 | ≤ 10 mg/kg/min |
| Oxacillin | 100 | 100 | 15 mins |
| Penicillin G | 1 million U/ml | Infants, 50,000 U/ml; Children, 100,000 U/ml | 15–30 mins |
| Pentamidine | 6 | 2.5 | 60 mins |
| Rifampin | 6 | 3 | 1–2 hrs |
| Ticarcillin (± clavulanate) | 100 | 50 | 15–30 mins |
| Tobramycin | 40 | 40 | 30 mins |
| Trimethoprim/sulfamethoxazole | 1.6 mg TMP | 1 mg TMP | 60 mins |
| Vancomycin | 5 | 5 | 1–2 hrs |
| Zidovudine | 4 | 4 | 60 mins |

## XIV. MAXIMUM DOSAGES FOR LARGE CHILDREN

Infants and young children have a large volume of distribution of many antibiotics in the body. Therefore, in order to achieve good serum concentrations, we give larger doses based on body weight or surface area than we give to adults. The following dosages of commonly used drugs are exceeded only in special circumstances. (See p. 95 for oral therapy of serious infections.)

| Maximum Daily Dosage | Antimicrobials |
|---|---|
| **ORAL FORMULATIONS** | |
| 4–8 g | Sulfisoxazole |
| 2–3 g | Amoxicillin, ampicillin, carbenicillin, cephalexin, cephradine, cloxacillin, nafcillin, oxacillin, penicillin G or V, tetracycline |
| 1–2 g | Cefaclor, cefprozil, cefuroxime axetil, ciprofloxacin, clindamycin, dicloxacillin, erythromycin, metronidazole |
| 0.5–1.2 g | Loracarbef, trimethoprim |
| 400 mg | Cefixime, cefpodoxime |
| **PARENTERAL FORMULATIONS** | |
| 18–24 g | Azlocillin, mezlocillin, piperacillin, ticarcillin |
| 10–12 g | Ampicillin, cefotaxime, ceftizoxime, cephalothin, methicillin, nafcillin, oxacillin |
| 6–8 g | Aztreonam, ceftazidime |
| 4–6 g | Cefamandole, cefazolin, cefuroxime, imipenem, meropenem |
| 2–4 g | Cefepime, ceftriaxone, chloramphenicol, clindamycin, erythromycin, metronidazole, spectinomycin, vancomycin |
| 1–2 g | Amikacin, cefonicid, ceforanide, streptomycin |
| 0.75–1.00 g | Kanamycin |
| 500 mg | Gentamicin, netilmicin, tobramycin |
| 20 million U | Penicillin G |
| 4.8 million U | Penicillin G, procaine |
| 2.4 million U | Penicillin G, benzathine |

## XV. DOSAGES BASED ON BODY SURFACE AREA

Antibiotic dosages calculated on the basis of body weight are not always appropriate for obese and malnourished patients. (Obese patients have excessively high serum concentrations; malnourished patients have lower than desired serum concentrations.) For such patients dosages calculated from body surface area are preferred. Infants usually have a greater body surface area than older children, although they also have greater antibiotic excretory ability than older children, allowing dosages based on weight to be acceptable for the majority of children, regardless of age.

Estimate body surface area (BSA) from nomograms available in many textbooks, or calculate it from the following formula:

$$\text{BSA (m}^2) = \text{wt (kg)}^{0.5378} \times \text{ht (cm)}^{0.3964} \times 0.024265$$

| Antibiotics (IM or IV) | Each Dose/m$^2$ | Interval | Amount/m$^2$/24 hrs |
|---|---|---|---|
| **Aminoglycoside** | | | |
| Amikacin, kanamycin | 200 mg | q8h | 600 mg |
| gentamicin, netilmicin, tobramycin | 60 mg | q8h | 180 mg |
| **Beta-Lactams** | | | |
| Penicillin G (meningitis) | 1,750,000 U | q4h | 10,500,000 U |
| Penicillin G (others) | 450,000 U | q4h | 2,700,000 U |
| Ampicillin, methicillin, oxacillin, cephalothin | 1.4 g | q6h | 5.6 g |
| Ceftriaxone | 1.4 g | q12h | 2.8 g |
| Ceftazidime | 1.4 g | q8h | 4.2 g |
| Nafcillin, cefamandole, cefotaxime, ceftizoxime | 1.05 g | q6h | 4.2 g |
| Cefazolin, cefuroxime | 0.8 g | q8h | 2.4 g |
| Cefonicid, ceforanide | 0.55 g | q12h | 1.1 g |
| Carbenicillin | 4 g | q6h | 16 g |
| Ticarcillin, azlocillin, mezlocillin, piperacillin | 2.5 g | q6h | 10 g |

| Antibiotics (IM or IV) | Each Dose/$m^2$ | Interval | Amount/$m^2$/24 hrs |
|---|---|---|---|
| Aztreonam | 0.8 g | q6h | 3.2 g |
| Imipenem | 0.55 g | q6h | 2.2 g |
| **Miscellaneous** | | | |
| Chloramphenicol (meningitis) | 0.7 g | q6h | 2.8 g |
| Chloramphenicol (others) | 0.45 g | q6h | 1.8 g |
| Metronidazole | 280 mg | q8h | 840 mg |
| Sulfamethoxazole | 0.5 g | q8h | 1.5 g |
| Trimethoprim | 100 mg | q8h | 300 mg |
| Vancomycin (CNS infection) | 0.425 g | q6h | 1.7 g |
| Vancomycin (others) | 0.275 g | q6h | 1.1 g |

## XVI. ADVERSE REACTIONS TO ANTIMICROBIAL AGENTS

A good rule of clinical practice is to be suspicious of an adverse drug reaction when a patient's clinical course deviates from the expected. This section focuses on reactions that require close observation or laboratory monitoring either because of their frequency or because of their severity. For detailed listings of reactions, consult the package inserts.

**Beta-Lactam Antibiotics.** The most feared reaction to penicillins, anaphylactic shock, is extremely rare, and no absolutely reliable means of predicting its occurrence exists. The commercially available skin testing material, benzyl-penicilloylpolylysine (Pre-Pen®), should be used in conjunction with the Minor Determinant Mixture (MDM) and penicilloic acid skin testing, but the latter two are not commercially available. A dilute solution of penicillin G (10,000 U/ml) can be used as a skin test material in place of MDM. If the scratch test and intradermal test with 0.01 ml are negative, penicillin of the same lot number should be used for administration to the patient. (Be prepared to treat anaphylaxis.) If the allergic status is questionable one can use a desensitization schedule (see Section X). The monobactam, aztreonam, does not exhibit cross-sensitization with penicillins and cephalosporins.

Ampicillin and other aminopenicillins cause minor adverse effects frequently. Oral or diaper area candidiasis, diarrhea, and morbilliform, and blotchy "ampicillin rashes" are common. The latter is not allergic in origin and is not a contraindication to subsequent use of ampicillin or any other penicillin. Diarrhea is somewhat less common with amoxicillin and more common with Augmentin®, but the new 7:1 formulation of Augmentin causes less diarrhea than the original formulation did. Rarely beta-lactams cause serious, life-threatening pseudomembranous enterocolitis due to suppression of normal bowel flora and overgrowth with *C. difficile*. Drug fever is probably more common with ampicillin than with other penicillins. Serum sickness is uncommon. Pancytopenia is rare, and reversible neutropenia and thrombocytopenia occasionally occur with any of the beta-lactams.

Nephrotoxicity is probably most common with methicillin (approximately 5%) but has been reported with all the penicillins (rarest with nafcillin). Hemorrhagic cystitis occurs mainly in poorly hydrated patients receiving large dosages and is probably a direct irritant effect of the large concentrations of drug in urine. It disappears even with continued use of the antibiotic when the patient's urine output increases. Ticarcillin interferes with platelet function but generally does not cause clinical bleeding problems. Hypokalemia with ticarcillin is more common than with other beta-lactams. Mezlocillin and piperacillin appear to have similar adverse effects to ticarcillin with the exception that mezlocillin has the least effect on platelet function.

Imipenem-cilastatin has similar adverse effects to other beta-lactams. In addition, patients occasionally have CNS reactions (convulsions, hallucinations, altered affect). Convulsions are most likely in the elderly or in patients with CNS disease, especially neonates. Meropenem does not have the undesirable CNS effects seen with imipenem.

The cephalosporins for oral use are generally better tolerated than the penicillins. The cephalosporins can cause a direct Coombs' reaction in the blood, but this is of no known clinical significance. Most cephalosporins are painful on IM injection and can cause phlebothrombosis with IV administration. Cefazolin and cefuroxime are better tolerated IM, and cefamandole and cephradine appear to cause fewer problems on IV use than the others. Cefaclor has been associated with a transient serum sickness–like reaction (rash, arthralgia); the cause is unknown. Similarly, a serum sickness–like reaction has been reported with IV use of cephapirin. Cefoperazone and cefamandole can cause a disulfiram (Antabuse)-like effect; patients should avoid alcohol, including elixirs. Prolonged prothrombin time and bleeding episodes have also been attributed to those drugs. It is treatable, and probably preventable, with vitamin K. The third generation cephalosporins cause profound alteration of normal flora on mucosal surfaces, and all have caused pseudomembranous colitis on rare occasions. Ceftriaxone commonly causes loose stools, but it is rarely severe enough to require stopping therapy. Ceftriaxone can cause sludging in the gallbladder (a calcium complex of ceftriaxone) that, on rare occasions, cause symptoms and jaundice; this is reversible after stopping the drug. Ceftriaxone is also reported to displace bilirubin from albumin-binding sites.

**Aminoglycosides.** Any of the aminoglycosidic aminocyclitol antibiotics can cause serious nephrotoxicity and ototoxicity. (The closely related aminocyclitol, spectinomycin, is safer in this respect.) The newer aminoglycosides (amikacin, tobramycin, gentamicin, and netilmicin) are generally safer than kanamycin, streptomycin or neomycin. In animal studies, netilmicin is the least ototoxic. Monitor all patients receiving aminoglycoside therapy for renal toxicity with periodic urinalyses and determinations of the BUN and creatinine and be alert to ototoxicity. Common practice is to measure the serum concentration 0.5–1 hour after a dose to make sure one is in a safe and therapeutic range and to measure a trough serum concentration immediately preceding a dose. Monitoring is especially important in patients with any degree of renal insufficiency. Elevated trough concentrations (> 2 μg/ml for gentamicin, netilmicin, and tobramycin, and > 10 μg/ml for amikacin and kanamycin) should be avoided. (With once daily administration regimens, peak values are two to three times greater.) Aminoglycosides potentiate botulinum toxin.

The "loop" diuretics (ethacrynic acid, furosemide, piretanide, and bumetanide) potentiate the ototoxicity of the aminoglycosides. The "non-loop" diuretics (hydrodiuril, mercuhydrin, and mannitol) do not interact with aminoglycosides to produce ototoxicity. Nephrotoxicity may be less common with once daily (as opposed to three times daily) dosing regimens.

The aminoglycosides are well tolerated via IM and IV routes of administration. Minor side effects, such as rashes and drug fever, are rare.

**Chloramphenicol.** The most feared toxicity of chloramphenicol, irreversible aplastic anemia, is very rare. It has been said that aplastic anemia is more likely with oral than with parenteral chloramphenicol, but documenting that claim is difficult, and it is probably incorrect. Regardless of the route of administration, laboratory monitoring for hematologic toxicity should be carried out in patients treated with chloramphenicol. Transient pharmacologic bone marrow depression occurs in almost all patients receiving large dosages (> 75 mg/kg per day) of chloramphenicol. As long as the absolute neutrophil count remains more than 1,500/l and the platelet count above 100,000/l, one can continue to administer chloramphenicol if it is necessary. These hematologic changes reverse rapidly when the drug is stopped.

The "gray syndrome" with potentially fatal circulatory collapse is due to excessive accumulation of chloramphenicol in neonates secondary to delayed conjugation (because of inadequate glucuronyl transferase activity) and poor renal excretion of unconjugated chloramphenicol. Chloramphenicol should not be used in neonates unless there are no suitable alternative drugs; dosage must be restricted and, ideally, one should monitor serum concentrations (therapeutic range 10–25 g/ml). Phenobarbital induces glucuronidative enzymes so that patients receiving phenobarbital may require larger-than-normal dosages of chloramphenicol. Rifampin has a similar effect. Concomitant phenytoin administration often causes accumulation of chloramphenicol in serum, which may reach a toxic concentration; conversely, accumulation of phenytoin to toxic concentrations has also been reported. Other drugs metabolized by the liver, such as theophylline, acetaminophen, and isoniazid, could have similar effects.

Minor side effects such as nausea and diarrhea are rare. With prolonged use (principally in children with cystic fibrosis), optic neuritis and peripheral neuritis have occurred. Alteration of normal respiratory and gastrointestinal flora may lead to infection with opportunistic bacteria or fungi. Drug fever is rare.

**Tetracyclines.** Tetracyclines are used infrequently in pediatric patients because the major indications are uncommon diseases (rickettsial infections, brucellosis), with the exception of acne, chlamydial infections, and Lyme disease. Side effects include minor gastrointestinal disturbances, photosensitization, angioedema, browning of the tongue, glossitis, pruritus ani, and exfoliative dermatitis. The diarrhea associated with tetracycline administration may be a direct irritant effect or due to alteration of normal GI flora with overgrowth of opportunistic bacteria or fungi. Alterations in normal respiratory tract flora produced by tetracycline increase the risk of superinfections by staphylococci and other opportunistic organisms.

Toxic effects from tetracyclines involve virtually every organ system. Hepatic and pancreatic injury have occurred with accidental overdosage and in patients with renal failure. (Pregnant women are particularly at risk for hepatic injury.) Tetracyclines are deposited in growing bones and teeth with depression of linear bone growth, dental staining, and defects in enamelization in deciduous and permanent teeth. This effect is dose-related and the risk extends up to 8 years of age. Patients taking outdated, degraded tetracycline can develop a Fanconi renal syndrome. Pseudotumor cerebri of unknown cause has rarely been seen in young infants who receive normal therapeutic doses. Minocycline causes dose-related vestibular toxicity in adults. Tetracycline is painful and irritative when injected into muscle, and thrombophlebitis occurs if the drug is given IV too rapidly.

**Macrolides.** Erythromycin is one of the safest antimicrobial agents. It commonly produces nausea and epigastric distress at dosages greater than 40 mg/kg/day. Decreased hearing that returns to normal after discontinuation of the drug has been reported. Alteration of normal flora is generally not a problem, but oral or perianal candidiasis occasionally develops. Transient cholestatic hepatitis is a rare complication that occurs with approximately equal frequency among the various formulations of erythromycin, but the estolate is said to pose a particular risk to pregnant women. Intramuscular administration of erythromycin is painful and irritative. Intravenous doses should be administered slowly (1–2 hours).

Clindamycin and lincomycin can cause nausea, vomiting, and diarrhea. Pseudomembranous colitis due to suppression of normal flora and overgrowth of *C. difficile* is uncommon, especially in children, but potentially serious. Urticaria, glossitis, pruritus and skin rashes occur occasionally. Serum sickness, anaphylaxis and photosensitivity are rare, as are hematologic and hepatic abnormalities.

The newer macrolides, azithromycin and clarithromycin, are less likely than erythromycin to cause gastrointestinal side effects.

**Polymyxins.** Polymyxin B and polymyxin E (colistin sulfate and colistimethate, respectively) are mainly of historic interest and are rarely used now except in topical preparations. With parenteral administration the major toxicity is to the kidneys. They also cause various neurological reactions such as flushing, dizziness, ataxia, diplopia, dysphagia, and paresthesias. Neuromuscular blockade with respiratory arrest has occurred. Hematologic or hepatic toxicity has rarely been attributed to the polymyxins. Oral colistin sulfate is well tolerated with few side effects.

**Antituberculous Drugs.** Isoniazid is generally well tolerated and hypersensitivity reactions are rare. Peripheral neuritis (preventable or reversed by pyridoxine administration) and mental aberrations from euphoria to psychosis occur more often in adults than in children. Mild elevations of ALT in the first weeks of therapy, which disappear with continued administration, are common. Rarely, frank hepatitis develops. Rifampin also can cause hepatitis; it is more common in patients with pre-existing liver disease or in those taking large dosages. Risk of hepatic damage increases when rifampin and isoniazid are taken together in dosages more than 15 mg/kg of each daily. Gastrointestinal, hematologic, and neurologic side effects of various types have been observed on occasion. Hypersensitivity reactions are rare. Pyrazinamide can cause hepatic damage, which appears to be dose-related. Ethambutol has the potential for ocular damage.

**Antifungal Drugs.** Amphotericin B, flucytosine, miconazole, ketoconazole, and itraconazole can produce serious adverse reactions. Amphotericin B is probably the most toxic antimicrobial drug in clinical use. Chills, fever, flushing, and headaches are the most common of the many adverse reactions. Some degree of decreased renal function occurs in as many as 80% of patients given amphotericin B. Anemia is common and, rarely, hepatic toxicity and neutropenia occur. Patients should be monitored for hypokalemia and hyponatremia. The lipid/liposomal formulations of amphotericin B probably cause less toxicity even though the daily dosages are larger.

The major toxicity of flucytosine is bone marrow depression, which is dosage-related, especially in patients treated concomitantly with amphotericin B. It also occurs in patients with a pre-existing hematologic disorder and in those treated with irradiation or cancer chemotherapeutic drugs. Mild gastrointestinal upset, mental confusion, and vertigo sometimes occur. Renal function should be monitored.

There has been little experience with the parenteral preparation of miconazole in children but it appears to be only slightly less toxic than amphotericin B. Patients receiving miconazole should be monitored for hematologic, hepatic, and renal toxicity.

Ketoconazole produces hepatic damage on rare occasions. The most common side effect is gastric distress; this can often be alleviated by dividing the daily dose. Gynecomastia is not rare in adult males. Itraconazole has a smaller incidence of adverse effects than ketoconazole.

Fluconazole is usually well tolerated. Gastrointestinal symptoms, rash, and headache occur occasionally. Transient, asymptomatic elevations of hepatic enzymes have been reported.

**Vancomycin.** Vancomycin can cause phlebitis if the drug is injected rapidly or in concentrated form. Vancomycin is said to have the potential for ototoxicity and nephrotoxicity, but documenting that these effects occur in children is difficult. It was reported that vancomycin potentiated the nephrotoxicity of aminoglycosides but further study showed that this was probably incorrect. Hepatic toxicity is rare. Neutropenia has been reported. If the drug is infused too rapidly, a transient rash of the upper body with itching may occur from histamine release ("red man syndrome"). It is not a contraindication to continued use and is less likely if the infusion rate is 60–120 minutes. Vancomycin in conjunction with anesthesia has been reported to cause hypotension and hypothermia.

**Sulfonamides and Trimethoprim.** The most common adverse reaction to sulfonamides is a hypersensitivity rash. Rarely, Stevens-Johnson syndrome occurs; it was most common with very long-acting sulfas that are no longer marketed. The frequency and types of reactions to the TMP/SMX combination are said to be the same as with sulfamethoxazole alone, but it is not clear whether Stevens-Johnson syndrome is caused more often by the combination than by sulfamethoxazole alone. Neutropenia and anemia occur occasionally. The rash caused by TMP/SMX appears to be more frequent in patients taking large dosages. Rash is common in adults with AIDS. Mild depression of platelet counts occurs in approximately one-half the patients treated with sulfas or TMP/SMX, but this rarely produces clinical bleeding problems. Sulfa drugs can precipitate hemolysis in patients with glucose-6-phosphate dehydrogenase deficiency. Crystalline aggregates of sulfa drugs may be deposited in the kidneys or ureters and cause acute nephropathy (most likely with sulfadiazine). Adequate urine output and alkalinization of the urine minimize the risk. Drug fever and serum sickness are infrequent hypersensitivity reactions.

Hepatitis with focal or diffuse necrosis is rare. A rare idiosyncratic reaction to sulfa drugs is acute aseptic meningitis.

**Fluoroquinolones.** All quinolone and fluoroquinolone drugs cause cartilage damage in toxicity studies in various immature animals; however, no conclusive data indicate similar toxicity in young children. Studies to evaluate this have, to date, not found cartilage toxicity in children. Reported side effects include gastrointestinal symptoms, dizziness, headaches, tremors, confusion, seizures, and rash. Hepatic toxicity is rare but appears to be more common with trovafloxacin than with the others. This fact limits the usefulness of trovafloxacin. Large dosages may precipitate hypoglycemia in the elderly.

**Antiviral Drugs.** After extensive clinical use, acyclovir has proved to be a safe drug with rare serious adverse effects. Renal dysfunction has occurred mainly with too rapid infusion of the drug. Rash, headache, and gastrointestinal side effects are uncommon. There has been no controlled experience in children with the related drugs, famciclovir, and valacyclovir.

Amantadine produces dizziness, drowsiness, and insomnia in many patients, but these effects are usually not severe. Visual disturbances, confusion, and psychosis are rare.

Foscarnet can cause renal dysfunction, anemia, and cardiac rhythm disturbances. Seizures and neuropathy are other serious but rare toxicities. Ganciclovir causes hematologic toxicity. Gastrointestinal disturbances and neurologic damage are rarely encountered.

The many antiviral drugs for treatment for HIV infection have many adverse effects; consult the package inserts.

# XVII. ADVERSE INTERACTIONS OF DRUGS

| Antibiotic | Interacting Drug | Adverse Effect |
| --- | --- | --- |
| Acyclovir | Probenecid | Poss incr acyclovir toxicity |
| Amantadine | Anticholinergics | Hallucinations, nightmares, confusion |
| Amikacin | (See Aminoglycosides) | |
| Aminoglycosides | Amphotericin B | Incr nephrotoxicity |
| | Anti-*Pseudomonas* penicillins (if renal failure) | Decr aminoglycoside serum conc |
| | Cephalosporins, cisplatin, cyclosporine | Poss incr nephrotoxicity |
| | Digoxin | Poss decr digoxin effect |
| | Ethacrynic acid, furosemide, bumetanide | Incr ototoxicity |
| | Indomethacin | Poss incr nephrotoxicity |
| | Methotrexate | Poss incr methotrexate toxicity |
| | Neuromuscular blocking agents; magnesium sulfate | Incr neuromuscular blockage |
| | Tacrolimus | Poss incr nephrotoxicity |
| Amphotericin B | Aminoglycosides | Incr nephrotoxicity |
| | Curariform drugs | Incr curariform effect |
| | Cyclosporine | Incr cyclosporine effect |
| | Digitalis drugs | Incr digitalis toxicity |
| | Miconazole | Decr anti-*Candida* effect |
| | Neuromuscular blocking agents | Hypokalemia |
| Ampicillin | Oral contraceptives | Decr contraceptive effect |
| | Allopurinol | Incr incidence of rash |

| Antibiotic | Interacting Drug | Adverse Effect |
|---|---|---|
| Cephalosporins | Alcohol (cefamandole, cefoperazone, moxalactam) | Antabuse-like effect |
| | Aminoglycosides | Poss incr nephrotoxicity |
| | Ethacrynic acid, furosemide | Incr nephrotoxicity |
| | Aspirin, heparin (moxalactam) | Poss incr bleeding risk |
| | Anticoagulants (moxalactam) | Incr anticoagulant effect |
| Chloramphenicol | Acetaminophen | Incr chloramphenicol toxicity |
| | Barbiturates | Incr barbiturate effect; Decr chloramphenicol effect |
| | Dicumarol | Incr anticoagulant effect |
| | Phenytoin | Altered pharmacology of both drugs |
| | Rifampin | Decr chloramphenicol effect |
| Ciprofloxacin | Theophylline, cyclosporine | Incr theophylline, cyclosporine |
| | Antacids | Decr ciprofloxacin absorption |
| Clarithromycin | (See Erythromycins) | |
| Clindamycin, Lincomycin | Neuromuscular blocking agents | Incr neuromuscular blockade |
| | Diphenoxylate-atropine | Incr diarrhea, colitis |
| Cycloserine | (See Isoniazid) | |
| Erythromycin | Anticoagulants | Incr anticoagulant effect |
| | Digoxin | Incr digoxin effect |
| | Theophylline | Incr theophylline effect |

| Antibiotic | Interacting Drug | Adverse Effect |
|---|---|---|
| | Carbamazepine | Incr carbamazepine effect |
| | Astemizole, cisapride | Cardiotoxicity |
| | Cyclosporine | Incr cyclosporine effect |
| Furazolidone | Alcohol | Antabuse-like effect |
| | Alpha-adrenergic amines | Incr hypertensive effect |
| Gentamicin | (See Aminoglycosides) | |
| Griseofulvin | Oral anticoagulants | Decr anticoagulant effect |
| | Phenobarbital | Decr griseofulvin effect |
| Intraconazole | (See Ketoconazole) | |
| Isoniazid | Aluminum antacids | Decr isoniazid effect |
| | Anticoagulants | Poss incr anticoagulant effect |
| | Carbamazepine | Incr toxicity of both drugs |
| | Cycloserine | Dizziness, drowsiness |
| | Phenytoin | Incr phenytoin toxicity |
| | Rifampin | Incr hepatotoxicity |
| Kanamycin | (See Aminoglycosides) | |
| Ketoconazole | Antacids, carbamazepine, cimetidine, didanosine, rifampin, phenytoin, phenobarbitol | Decr ketoconazole effect |
| | Cisapride | Cardiotoxicity |
| | Cyclosporine | Incr cyclosporine effect |
| | Erythromycin | Cardiotoxicity |
| | Tacrolimus | Incr tacrolimus effect |
| Lincomycin | (See Clindamycin) | |

| Antibiotic | Interacting Drug | Adverse Effect |
|---|---|---|
| Metronidazole | Alcohol | Antabuse-like reaction |
| | Anticoagulants | Incr anticoagulant effect |
| | Phenobarbital | Decr metronidazole effect |
| Miconazole | (See Amphotericin B) | |
| Nalidixic acid | Oral anticoagulants | Incr anticoagulant effect |
| Netilmicin | (See Aminoglycosides) | |
| Quinacrine | Alcohol | Antabuse-like effect |
| Rifampin | Anticoagulants, barbiturates, beta-adrenergic blockers, contraceptives, corticosteroids, cyclosporine, diazepam, digitoxin, hypoglycemics, tacrolimus, quinidine | Decreased effect of interacting drug |
| | Chloramphenicol | Decr chloramphenicol effect |
| | Isoniazid | Incr hepatotoxicity |
| | Methadone | Methadone withdrawal symptoms |
| Spectinomycin | Lithium | Incr lithium toxicity |
| Streptomycin | (See Aminoglycosides) | |
| | Cyclosporine | Decr cyclosporine effect |
| Sulfonamides | Oral anticoagulants | Incr anticoagulant effect |
| | Cyclosporine | Decr cyclosporine effect |
| | Hypoglycemics | Incr hypoglycemia |
| | Methotrexate | Poss incr methotrexate toxicity |
| | Phenytoin | Incr phenytoin effect |
| | Thiopental | Incr thiopental effect |

| Antibiotic | Interacting Drug | Adverse Effect |
|---|---|---|
| Tetracyclines | Antacids, bismuth subsalicylate, iron, zinc sulfate | Decr tetracycline effect |
| | Phenytoin, barbiturates and carbamazepine | Decr doxycycline effect |
| | Oral contraceptives | Decr contraceptive effect |
| | Lithium | Incr lithium toxicity |
| Thiabendazole | Theophylline | Incr theophylline effect |
| Tobramycin | (See Aminoglycosides) | |

Conc, concentration; Decr, decrease; Incr, increase; Poss, possible.

# XVIII. INDEX OF DISEASES